Essential MCQs
in
Obstetrics and Gynaecology
for
Medical Students

Diana Hamilton-Fairley MD FRCOG
Consultant Obstetrician and Gynaecologist
Deputy Director of Postgraduate
Medical Education
Guys and St. Thomas' NHS Trust
London

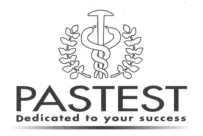

PASTEST
Dedicated to your success

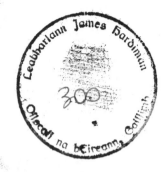

© 2003 PasTest Ltd
Egerton Court
Parkgate Estate
Knutsford
Cheshire
WA16 8DX

Telephone: 01565 752000

First published 2003

ISBN 1 901198 34 0

A catalogue record for this book is available from the British Library.

The information contained within this book was obtained by the author from reliable sources. However, while every effort has been made to ensure its accuracy, no responsibility for loss, damage or injury occasioned to any person acting or refraining from action as a result of information contained herein can be accepted by the publishers or author.

PasTest Revision Books and Intensive Courses

PasTest has been established in the field of postgraduate medical education since 1972, providing revision books and intensive study courses for doctors preparing for their professional examinations.

Books and courses are available for the following specialties:
MRCP Parts 1 and 2, MRCPCH Parts 1 and 2, MRCGP, MRCPsych, MRCS, MRCOG Parts 1 and 2, DRCOG, DCH, FRCA, PLAB Parts 1 and 2.

For further details contact:

PasTest Ltd, Freepost, Knutsford, Cheshire WA16 7BR
Tel: 01565 752000   Fax: 01565 650264
www.pastest.co.uk   enquiries@pastest.co.uk

Typeset by Breeze Limited, Manchester
Printed and bound by MPG Books Ltd, Bodmin, Cornwall

CONTENTS

INTRODUCTION

This book provides multiple choice questions (MCQs), extended matching questions (EMQs), and clinically applicable questions for medical students approaching their Obstetrics and Gynaecology examinations. In many medical schools the format of examinations for testing knowledge is changing and I hope this book provides some practise in these alternative formats.

The questions are all based on the core knowledge required in the medical curriculum. Some of the questions are deliberately harder than others so that you can explore the depths of your knowledge and understanding. The aim of this strategy is that if these practice papers seem hard then the exam itself will appear easier, giving you confidence to be sure of your answers in the real situation. This book gives three practice papers with answers and explanations at the end of each paper. The questions cover three main areas: basic science, obstetrics and gynaecology. Many of the questions have been seen and edited by current medical students who have found the format to be a good and rewarding way to revise. I hope you will agree.

I would like to thank two of my colleagues for their help in writing some questions, and advice on the setting of the new types of question, Dr Prabha Sinha, Consultant Obstetrician and Gynaecologist, Conquest Hospital, Hastings and Mr Michael Marsh, Senior Lecturer in Obstetrics and Gynaecology at King's College Hospital, London.

Diana Hamilton-Fairley

MCQ EXAMINATION TECHNIQUE

MCQ examinations are primarily used to test knowledge, although the new types of questions are beginning to test application of knowledge, in particular clinical scenarios. It is important for students to establish the exact nature of the examination and the following is a useful checklist:

- ✓ **How many questions are in the paper?**
- ✓ **How long does the examination last?**
- ✓ **What are the formats of the questions?**
- ✓ **Is the exam negatively marked, ie is a minus mark given for a wrong answer?** This can alter the way you approach the exam with many people saying that you should aim to answer at least 80% of the paper to stand a good chance of passing.
- ✓ **Will you be expected to interpret results from investigations and if so will normal values be provided?** If you will not be provided with normal values you need to learn the core ones in this book.
- ✓ **How is the answer paper structured?** They vary from university to university. There is a sample answer sheet on p.xi.
- ✓ **What is your university's preferred method for marking the answer paper?**
- ✓ **Are pencils and rubbers provided?** If not remember to take your own and if you have to mark the paper in pencil, remember to take a pencil sharpener also.

As with all examinations make sure that you have read the instructions on the answer sheet carefully and ensure your candidate number is correct.

Read the questions carefully. It is easy to skip through the stem and make assumptions about the nature of the question, only to find that the question contained a clue that you have missed. These include questions where only one answer is correct, although more than one of the possible answers may relate to the topic. Make sure you understand what the question is asking, eg is it asking you to identify the true or the false statements? Many candidates get confused by the words used in the stem by over analysis of what the words mean. MCQs are not easy to create and on the whole the examiners try to be very precise in their use of words but occasionally you have to use a general interpretation or instinct to know what the question is asking.

When you are looking at the possible answers treat each one individually, relating it back to the stem before making a decision. You can then mark the answer straight onto the answer sheet taking care to fill in the correct lozenge, block or square. If you use this approach it is a good idea to mark your answer on the paper as well so that you can go back and check that you have filled in the answer sheet correctly. Some students go through the paper and mark true/false on the paper and then transfer the answers to the answer sheet. This can lead to errors as it is repetitive and it is easy to lose your place on the answer sheet and put the wrong answers to the question by a transcription error.

It is very important that you fill in the answer sheet using the correct method – the papers are marked by computers that will not show any leniency towards even the smallest transgression in filling in the sheet. If the answer sheet has areas that say they should not be marked then make sure you do not inadvertently make a line, dot or doodle in them. This is because the computer will reject the whole paper - a very frustrating way to fail an exam that you might otherwise have passed.

When you have finished the exam by whichever method you choose it is wise to go back and check the answers. I recommend you use this time to check that the answer sheet is correctly filled, that no answers are obviously wrong and that you correctly understood the question. I learnt from bitter experience that changing more than one or two of my original answers usually made my mark lower rather than higher. When you start the paper your mind is fresh, by the end of the exam you are tired, so it is more likely that you will make foolish errors. Unless you are absolutely sure that the new answer is correct I would counsel making as few changes as possible – your first instinctive answer is more likely to be the correct one.

Revising for MCQ papers is best done using real practice papers or revision texts such as this one. This ensures that you cover the whole syllabus and identify your strengths and weaknesses.

This book can be used in many ways. The three practice papers can be used as timed practice papers. It is not easy to be disciplined when doing a paper at home with the answers readily available at the back but it is worth doing as it will give you a guide to areas that need further work before the exam. Timing yourself will tell you how fast you work and whether you can afford to slow down or need to speed up.

The index can be used to look for questions in a particular area so that you can check that a topic you have just revised is properly understood and retained.

You can use the book to revise in a group so that you can teach each other areas where one is weak and another strong. It is also more fun and often leads to a deepening of knowledge, understanding and application of that knowledge through discussion and often heated debate.

If you find a topic that you have struggled with then do not rely solely on the brief notes given with the answers. Guessing or having no idea means there is a gap in your knowledge which needs filling by reading round the subject from a textbook or your lecture/seminar notes.

SAMPLE ANSWER SHEET

UNIVERSITY OF LONDON Management Systems Division

MULTIPLE-CHOICE EXAMINATION ANSWER SHEET

	Candidate No.	Test No.	College No.

DATE..................

SURNAME..................

FIRST NAME(S)..................

Instructions: Use the HB pencil provided. To make an answer draw a single horizontal line along the dotted line above the appropriate letter or number. To answer 'TRUE' draw your line above the capital letter in the upper row. To answer 'FALSE' draw your line above the lower case letter in the lower row. For example:

[A] for 'TRUE'   [A] for 'FALSE'
[a]   [a]

If you change your mind and wish to cancel a completed answer, draw another line below the letter or number, along the dotted line. Do not rub out.

Candidate No. / Test No. / College No. number grids:

[0] [0] [0] [0]	[0] [0] [0] [0]	[0] [0]
[1] [1] [1] [1]	[1] [1] [1] [1]	[1] [1]
[2] [2] [2] [2]	[P] [2] [2] [2]	[2] [2]
[3] [3] [3] [3]	[3] [3] [3]	[3] [3]
[4] [4] [4] [4]	[4] [4] [4]	[4] [4]
[5] [5] [5] [5]	[5] [5] [5]	[5] [5]
[6] [6] [6] [6]	[6] [6] [6]	[6] [6]
[7] [7] [7] [7]	[7] [7] [7]	[7] [7]
[8] [8] [8] [8]	[8] [8] [8]	[8] [8]
[9] [9] [9] [9]	[9] [9] [9]	[9] [9]

Shown below is the correct method of completion, the correct method of cancellation/alteration and examples of various incorrect methods of completion.

CORRECT METHOD OF COMPLETION

True = [A]   False = [A]
       [a]   [a]

CORRECT METHOD OF CANCELLATION/ ALTERATION

To cancel a response, draw a line below the letter. Do not rub out. Thus:

[A] or [A] = Cancelled
[a]   [a]

To alter a response, first cancel. Then draw a line above the other letter. Thus:

False = [A]   True = [A]
        [a]   [a]

INCORRECT METHODS OF COMPLETION

Too faint [A]
Slanted [A]
Too low [A]
Too high [A]
Into next box [A] [B]
Too short [A] [A] [A]
Isolated cancellation [A]
DETERMINATE TYPE T

Answer grid (columns 1–60), each with rows A B C D E (upper) and a b c d e (lower):

1–12, 13–24, 25–36, 37–48, 49–60

Reproduced with kind permission of the University of London

x

ABBREVIATIONS

AC	Abdominal circumference
AFP	Alpha fetoprotein
Alb	Albumin
ALP	Alkaline phosphatase
ALT	Alanine transaminase
ARM	Artificial rupture of membranes
AST	Aspartate transaminase
βhCG	Beta-human chorionic gonadotrophin
Bili	Bilirubin
BMI	Body mass index (wt (kg)/height $(m)^2$)
BP	Blood pressure
BPM	Beats per minute
BV	Bacterial vaginosis
CEA	Coelomic embryonic antigen
CHD	Congenital heart disease
CIN	Cervical intraepithelial neoplasia
CL	Corpus luteum
CNS	Central nervous system
COCP	Combined oral contraceptive pill
CRP	C-reactive protein
CT	Computerised tomography
CTG	Cardiotocograph
CVS	Chorionic villus sampling
DI	Detrusor instability
DMPA	Depomedroxyprogesterone acetate
DUB	Dysfunctional uterine bleeding
E2	Oestradiol
ECG	Electrocardiograph
ECV	External cephalic version
EDD	Expected date of delivery
ELISA	Enzyme-linked immunoabsorbant assay
FBC	Full blood count
FSH	Follicle stimulating hormone
GDM	Gestational diabetes mellitus
GGT	Gamma-glutamyl transpeptidase
GnRH	Gonadotrophin releasing hormone
GSUI	Genuine stress urinary incontinence
Hb	Haemoglobin
HbA	Adult haemoglobin
HbS	Sickle cell haemoglobin

Abbreviations

HC	Head circumference
HcG	Human chorionic gonadotrophin
HELLP syndrome	Haemolysis, elevated liver enzymes, low platelets
HIV	Human immunodeficiency virus
HPV	Human papilloma virus
HSV	Herpes simplex virus
ICSI	Intracytoplasmic sperm injection
IDDM	Insulin dependent diabetes mellitus (type 1)
IgA	Immunoglobin A
IgG	Immunoglobin G
IGT	Impaired glucose tolerance
IOL	Induction of labour
IUCD	Intrauterine contraceptive device
IUD	Intrauterine death
IUGR	Intrauterine growth restriction (ex. retardation)
IUS	Intrauterine system
L/S ratio	Lecithin / sphingomyelin ratio
LDH	Lactate dehydrogenase
LETZ	Loop excision of the transformation zone
LH	Luteinising hormone
LMP	Last menstrual period
LSCS	Lower segment Caesarean section
M, C & S	Microscopy, culture and sensitivity
MCV	Mean corpuscular volume
MRI	Magnetic resonance imaging
MSAFP	Maternal serum alpha fetoprotein
NICE	National Institute of Clinical Excellence
NIDDM	Non-insulin dependent diabetes mellitus (type 2)
NSAIDs	Non-steroidal anti-inflammatory drugs
NTD	Neural tube defect
OCP	Oral contraceptive pill
OGTT	Oral glucose tolerance test
P	Progesterone
PCOS	Polycystic ovary syndrome
PCR	Polymerase chain reaction
PCV	Packed cell volume
PET	Pre-eclamptic toxaemia
PID	Pelvic inflammatory disease
PIH	Pregnancy induced hypertension

Plts	Platelets
POP	Progestogen only pill
PPROM	Preterm premature rupture of membranes
PRL	Prolactin
RM	Recurrent miscarriage
RML	Right medio-lateral
RNA	Ribonucleic acid
SROM	Spontaneous rupture of membranes
T	Testosterone
T4	Thyroxine
TSH	Thyroid stimulating hormone
TPHA	Treponema pallidum haemagglutination test
TV	*Trichomonas vaginalis*
UA	Umbilical artery
USS	Ultrasound scan
UV	Umbilical vein
VaIN	Vaginal intraepithelial neoplasia
VDRL	Venereal disease research laboratory
VIN	Vulval intraepithelial neoplasia

NORMAL VALUES

Women

	Non-Pregnant	Pregnant
Haematology		
Hb	11.5–15.5 g/dl	10.5–13.5 g/dl
MCV	76–98 fl	
PCV	35–55%	30–45%
WCC	4-11 × 10^9/l	6–13 × 10^9/l
Plts	150–400 × 10^9/l	
Ferritin	15–120 µg/l	
Folate	1.5–10.0 µg/l	
Vitamin B$_{12}$	160–900 pmol/l	
Biochemistry		
Na	135–145 mmol/l	
K	3.5–5.0 mmol/l	
U	2.5–6.5 mmol/l	1.8–4.5 mmol/l
Creatinine	50–120 µmol/l	45–63 µmol/l
ALT	0–55 iu/l	
AST	10–40 iu/l	
Bilirubin	2–17 mmol/l	
ALP	30–130 iu/l	90–500 iu/l
Alb	35–55 g/l	20–45 g/l
GGT	5–30 iu/l	
Urate	0.1–0.4 mol/l	< 0.35 mol/l
CRP	< 7 mg/l	
Diabetes		
Random glucose	3.5–5.5 mmol/l	
OGTT at 2 hours	< 7.8 mmol/l normal	
	7.9–11 mmol/l IGT	
	>11 mmol/lDM	
Hb A1C	< 7.0%	
Endocrinology		
Prolactin	< 400 mu/l	
TSH	0.17–3.2 miu/l	
T4	11–22 pmol/l	

Follicle stimulating hormone (FSH)

Prepubertal children	< 5 iu/l
Follicular phase	2.5–10 iu/l
Mid-cycle	25–70 iu/l
Luteal phase	0.3–2 iu/l
Postmenopausal	> 20 iu/l

Luteinising hormone (LH)

Prepubertal children	<5 iu/l
Follicular phase	2.5–10 iu/l
Mid-cycle	25–70 iu/l
Luteal phase	0.5–13 iu/l
Postmenopausal	> 20 iu/l
Testosterone	0.5–2.4 nmol/l

Oestradiol

Prepubertal children	< 150 pmol/l
Follicular phase	150–450 pmol/l
Mid-cycle	600–1200 pmol/l
Luteal phase	150–450 pmol/l
Postmenopausal	< 150 pmol/l

Progesterone

Follicular phase	< 3 nmol/l
Mid-luteal phase	> 25 nmol/l indicates ovulation
Failing pregnancy	< 5 nmol/l

Tumour markers

Ca125	< 25 iu/l
Ca199	< 8 iu/l
CEA	< 8 iu/l
βhCG	< 25 iu/l > 25 iu/l
	visible pregnancy on USS > 1000 iu/l
	60% rise in 48 h = ongoing pregnancy
AFP	< 8 iu/l
LDH	286-580 II/l

Men

LH	1–8 iu/l
FSH	1–8 iu/l
Testosterone	9–30 nmol/l

Male Fertility Tests

Sperm count	$> 20 \times 10^6$/ml
Motility	> 50% actively motile
Morphology	> 10% normal forms
Volume	1.5–3 ml

Routine antenatal booking blood tests
FBC
Haemoglobinopathy screen
Blood group
HIV screening
Syphilis screening (VDRL / TPHA)
Rubella immunity
Hepatitis B screening

Down's syndrome screening

USS — Nuchal thickness > 3 mm 11–13 weeks
Serum screening

βhCG
AFP   } Risk > 1:250 considered high risk
Oestriol

DEFINITIONS COMMONLY TESTED IN MCQ PAPERS

Total Birth rate
Births per year × 1000/midyear population

General fertility rate
Births per year × 1000/women aged from 15–45

Fetal viability
A fetus that is delivered after 24 completed weeks of pregnancy

Premature labour
Labour occurring before 37 completed weeks of pregnancy

Term pregnancy
A pregnancy that has lasted longer than 37 completed weeks of pregnancy

Maternal mortality
Deaths during pregnancy or within one year of delivery/1000 births or 100,000 maternities

Perinatal mortality
Number of stillbirths + deaths within 7 days/1000 births

Pregnancy induced hypertension
A > 15 mmHg rise in the diastolic blood pressure from booking BP on two occasions

Pre-eclamptic toxaemia (PET)
A > 15 mmHg rise in the diastolic blood pressure from booking BP on two occasions with significant proteinuria (> 300 mg/24 h)

Pearl index (for methods of contraception)
Number of pregnancies × 100/number of couples using the method

Dysfunctional uterine bleeding (DUB)
Excessive menstrual loss associated with no proven pathology

Genuine stress urinary incontinence (GSUI)
Involuntary loss of urine when the transmitted intra-abdominal pressure causes a rise in the intravesical pressure that exceeds the intraurethral pressure in the absence of detrusor contractions

Menopause
Absence of menses for greater than one calendar year associated with a rise in follicle stimulating hormone

Primary amenorrhoea
1. A girl of 14 who has never had a period in the absence of secondary sexual characteristics
2. A girl of 16 who has never had a period in the presence of secondary sexual characteristics

Secondary amenorrhoea
The absence of menses for greater than six months in a woman who has previously had periods

Primary subfertility
A person/couple who has/have never conceived after one year of regular unprotected sexual intercourse

Secondary subfertility
A person/couple who have conceived in the past but have failed to conceive after one year of regular unprotected sexual intercourse

Early miscarriage
The spontaneous loss of a pregnancy before 12 completed weeks of pregnancy

Late miscarriage
The spontaneous loss of a pregnancy beyond 12 completed weeks of pregnancy and before 24 completed weeks of pregnancy

Recurrent miscarriage
The spontaneous loss of three or more pregnancies before 24 completed weeks of pregnancy

Definitions commonly tested in MCQ papers

Bishop's Score	0	1	2
Cervical length	> 2 cm	1–2 cm	< 1 cm
Cervical position	Posterior	Mid	Anterior
Cervical dilatation	Closed	1 cm	> 2 cm
Cervical consistency	Firm	Med	Soft
Station of the head	-2 cm	-1 cm	At spines or below

Expected date of delivery (EDD)
LMP + 7 days – 3 months

PRACTICE PAPER 1

50 questions: Time allowed 2 hours.
Mark your answer with a tick (True) or a cross (False).
Do not look at the answers until you have completed the whole paper.
Answers and teaching notes are on page 21.

PRACTICE PAPER 1

1.1 **The principle supports of the uterus are**

- ❏ A the iliosacral ligaments
- ❏ B the pyriformis muscle
- ❏ C the transverse cervical ligaments
- ❏ D the infundibular ligaments
- ❏ E the uterosacral ligaments

1.2 **Which of the following statements are true?**

- ❏ A The ovary is attached to the lateral pelvic side-wall
- ❏ B The ureter lies beneath the uterine artery
- ❏ C The mucosa of the fallopian tube is lined by ciliated cells
- ❏ D The pouch of Douglas lies between the bladder and the uterus
- ❏ E The polar body of the oocyte contains 23 chromosomes

1.3 **A 46-year-old woman who has been happily married for 18 years complains of irregular vaginal bleeding. Which five of the following should be performed as first-line investigations?**

- ❏ A Full blood count
- ❏ B Urea and electrolytes
- ❏ C Cervical smear
- ❏ D Cervical swab for chlamydia
- ❏ E Transvaginal ultrasound scan
- ❏ F Hysteroscopy and endometrial biopsy
- ❏ G Endometrial biopsy
- ❏ H Speculum examination
- ❏ I Digital vaginal examination
- ❏ J Group and save

1.4   In a sagittal cross section of the pelvis

❏ A   the urethra lies anterior to the upper third of the vagina
❏ B   the urethra lies anterior to the lower third of the vagina
❏ C   the bladder when empty lies below and anterior to the uterine body
❏ D   the bladder when empty lies parallel and anterior to the uterine body
❏ E   the rectum lies posterior to the body of the uterus

1.5   Which of the following structures lie within the broad ligament?

❏ A   The fallopian tube
❏ B   The ureter
❏ C   The uterine artery
❏ D   The ovarian artery
❏ E   The superior vesical artery

1.6   Match the following A–E to five of the statements below.

During the menstrual cycle

A follicle stimulating hormone
B oestradiol
C progesterone
D testosterone
E the first meiotic division

❏ 1   is completed following the LH surge
❏ 2   is produced by the adrenal gland
❏ 3   is completed during the neonatal period
❏ 4   is inhibited by oestradiol
❏ 5   decreases mid-cycle
❏ 6   is a precursor of oestradiol
❏ 7   is inhibited by GnRH
❏ 8   is produced throughout the cycle
❏ 9   is produced in the secretory phase
❏ 10 is secreted by the hypothalamus

1.7 Complications of laparoscopy include perforation of the

❏ A gall bladder
❏ B urinary bladder
❏ C uterus
❏ D inferior vesical artery
❏ E inferior epigastric artery

1.8 In the follicular phase of the menstrual cycle

❏ A the granulosa cells produce androstenedione and testosterone
❏ B the endometrial glands become straight
❏ C oestradiol inhibits the production of LH
❏ D the thecal cells produce oestradiol and secrete follicular fluid
❏ E the nucleus of the oocyte contains 23 chromosomes

1.9 In embryo development

❏ A beta human chorionic gonadotrophin (βhCG) is produced by the fallopian tube from the moment of fertilisation
❏ B the blastocyst divides into two halves, one forming the embryo, the other the placenta
❏ C the villi of the developing embryo invade the maternal capillaries
❏ D the fetal heart starts beating at around five weeks from date of last menstrual period
❏ E haemoglobin F has a lesser affinity for oxygen than haemoglobin A

1.10 After birth which of the following changes occur in the fetus?

❏ A The foramen ovale closes allowing the entire blood volume to circulate into the pulmonary artery
❏ B Lung fluid is forced out of the fetal alveoli with the first few breaths
❏ C The ductus arteriosus opens
❏ D Haemoglobin F is replaced by haemoglobin A
❏ E The umbilical vein and artery remain open for several weeks

1.11 Mark as true the five best matched statements about βhCG:

❏ A βhCG begins to rise two weeks after fertilisation
❏ B βhCG is measured using a monoclonal antibody radioimmunoassay
❏ C It is a hormone secreted by the trophoblastic cells of the developing placenta
❏ D The β-subunit is the same as TSH and FSH
❏ E A low level of βhCG is associated with an increased risk of a baby with Down's syndrome
❏ F The half-life of βhCG in plasma is 96 hours
❏ G A high level of βhCG is associated with a hydatidiform mole
❏ H Serial βhCG measurements are useful in the diagnosis of an ectopic pregnancy
❏ I βhCG is a polypeptide protein produced by the hypothalamus
❏ J A high level of βhCG is associated with a multiple pregnancy

1.12 Which of the following statements are true about luteinising hormone (LH)/follicle stimulating hormone (FSH)?

❏ A They are glycoproteins
❏ B They are secreted continuously by the pituitary gland
❏ C LH stimulates the formation of the corpus luteum
❏ D LH and FSH increases in the middle of the cycle
❏ E The LH surge occurs in the middle of a 28 day cycle and lasts for three days

1.13 Mark as true the five best matched statements about the menopause:

❑ A   The current average age of menopause in the US is 51 years
❑ B   LH levels rise before FSH levels
❑ C   The ovaries become more resistant to the action of FSH
❑ D   FSH levels rise before LH levels
❑ E   Menopausal women are prone to vertebral crush fractures
❑ F   The risk of myocardial infarction is reduced in menopausal women
❑ G   Lack of oestrogen leads to osteopenia
❑ H   Variation in cycle lengths is more common around the time of the menopause
❑ I   High FSH levels cause hot flushes
❑ J   Menopausal women rarely complain of dyspareunia

1.14 A 26-year-old primigravid woman at ten weeks gestation visits her midwife for a routine booking appointment. She has sickle cell anaemia. Her partner's sickle cell status is HbAS. What are the chances of her baby having sickle cell disease?

❑ A   1 in 8
❑ B   1 in 4
❑ C   1 in 5
❑ D   1 in 2
❑ E   1 in 3

1.15 Which one of the following statements about amniotic fluid is correct?

❑ A   The volume of amniotic fluid has no prognostic value in pregnancy
❑ B   An increased amniotic fluid volume may be associated with fetal chromosomal abnormalities
❑ C   A decreased amniotic fluid volume may be associated with fetal chromosomal abnormalities
❑ D   Amniotic fluid is derived solely from the amnion at 36 weeks
❑ E   Amniotic fluid contains bilirubin in healthy pregnancies

1.16 Which of the following disorders are inherited as an autosomal dominant disorder?

- ❑ A Sickle cell disease
- ❑ B Duchenne muscular dystrophy
- ❑ C Haemophilia
- ❑ D Huntington's chorea
- ❑ E Cystic fibrosis

1.17 The greatest contribution to vaginal lubrication comes from

- ❑ A fluid from Skene's glands
- ❑ B mucus produced by endocervical glands
- ❑ C viscous fluid from Bartholin's glands
- ❑ D transudate-like material from the vaginal walls
- ❑ E the uterine wall

1.18 A woman presents to the Accident and Emergency department 15 days after giving birth by Caesarean section. She complains of persistent vaginal bleeding. Her temperature is 37.5°C, pulse 88 bpm and BP 110/76 mmHg. What is the most likely diagnosis?

- ❑ A Mastitis
- ❑ B Endometritis
- ❑ C Retained products of conception
- ❑ D Wound infection
- ❑ E Wound haematoma

1.19 Which of the following are normal vaginal commensals?

- ❑ A *Escherichia coli*
- ❑ B β Haemolytic streptococcus
- ❑ C *Candida albicans*
- ❑ D *Staphylococcus aureus*
- ❑ E Doderlein's bacilli

1.20 At each routine antenatal visit which of the following should be performed?

❏ A Vaginal examination
❏ B Blood pressure
❏ C Symphysiofundal height
❏ D Cardiotocography
❏ E Haemoglobin

1.21 Choose from the following five best matched statements about diabetes in pregnancy

❏ A Women who smoke are at increased risk of developing gestational diabetes mellitus (GDM)
❏ B Glucose is more commonly found in the urine of pregnant women than non-pregnant women
❏ C Poor glycaemic control in pre-pregnancy type 1 diabetes is associated with a two-fold increase in congenital abnormalities
❏ D Gestational diabetes commonly develops before 28 weeks gestation
❏ E Women with a first degree relative with type 2 diabetes should have a glucose tolerance test at 28 weeks
❏ F Macrosomia is associated with glucose concentrations of 4–7.8 mmol/l
❏ G GDM is associated with an increased risk of intrauterine death beyond 40 weeks gestation
❏ H Intrauterine growth restriction is associated with type 1 diabetes in the presence of maternal retinopathy and nephropathy
❏ I GDM is associated with a reduced risk of intrauterine death beyond 40 weeks gestation
❏ J Poor glycaemic control in pre-pregnancy type 1 diabetes is associated with a 3-fold increased risk in congenital abnormalities

1.22 Which of the following drugs are known to have a teratogenic potential?

- ❏ A Prednisolone
- ❏ B Danazol
- ❏ C Warfarin
- ❏ D Sodium valproate
- ❏ E ACE inhibitors

1.23 Pregnancy induced hypertension without proteinuria

- ❏ A is associated with intrauterine growth restriction
- ❏ B is associated with an increased risk of intrauterine death
- ❏ C is associated with cephalo-pelvic disproportion
- ❏ D can be safely treated with methyldopa
- ❏ E most commonly arises after the 37th completed week of gestation

1.24 Which of the following are common early signs of pregnancy?

- ❏ A Varicose veins
- ❏ B Urinary retention
- ❏ C Breast tenderness
- ❏ D Primary amenorrhoea
- ❏ E Nausea

1.25 Fetal echocardiography is indicated in

- ❏ A family history of cardiac anomaly
- ❏ B pre-existing maternal diabetes
- ❏ C exposure to phenytoin
- ❏ D fetal arrhythmia
- ❏ E fetal hydrops

1.26 **A 35-year-old multigravida had a maternal serum α-fetoprotein (MSAFP) screening test performed at 16 weeks in her current pregnancy (based on a dating scan at 11 weeks gestation). The result shows a significantly raised level. Which of the following is the most likely explanation for this finding?**

- ❏ A Open neural tube defect (NTD)
- ❏ B Abdominal wall defect
- ❏ C Wrong dates
- ❏ D Bleeding in early pregnancy
- ❏ E Fetal demise

1.27 **A 26-year-old woman in her second pregnancy at 28 weeks gestation comes to the antenatal clinic and is found to have a breech presentation. When should an external cephalic version (ECV) be attempted?**

- ❏ A At 30–31 weeks
- ❏ B At 37–39 weeks
- ❏ C At 34–36 weeks
- ❏ D At 32–33 weeks
- ❏ E At 40–41 weeks

1.28 **A 19-year-old woman at 38 weeks gestation in her first pregnancy attends the labour ward with intermittent abdominal pain. On vaginal examination the cervix is 1 cm dilated and 100% effaced and the fetal head is at the level of the ischial spines. Which of the following is the most likely diagnosis?**

- ❏ A Latent phase of labour
- ❏ B Active phase of labour
- ❏ C Transitional phase of labour
- ❏ D Third stage of labour
- ❏ E Second stage of labour

1.29 **A woman is admitted in spontaneous labour at term. She had a Caesarean section in her first pregnancy because the baby became distressed when she was 6 cm dilated. Which of the following are true?**

- ❏ A The risk of uterine rupture is 4–5%
- ❏ B The risk of uterine rupture is 1–2%
- ❏ C The risk of uterine rupture is 0.1–0.2%
- ❏ D The chances of achieving a vaginal birth are 70%
- ❏ E The chances of achieving a vaginal birth are 50%

1.30 **Which of the following are indications for an emergency lower segment Caesarean section in a woman who has had an uncomplicated pregnancy? She is 31 years old, in her first pregnancy and presented in spontaneous labour at 39 weeks. The CTG is normal and the liquor is clear. She has a working epidural and has been on Syntocinon for three hours for slow progress at 7 cm. She is now fully dilated.**

- ❏ A An occipito-posterior position one hour following full dilation with the fetal head 0/5 palpable per abdomen
- ❏ B An occipito-posterior position two hours following full dilation with the fetal head 0/5 palpable per abdomen
- ❏ C An occipito-posterior position two hours following full dilation with the fetal head 2/5 palpable per abdomen
- ❏ D An occipito-anterior position two hours following full dilation with the fetal head 0/5 palpable per abdomen
- ❏ E An occipito-anterior position two hours following full dilation with the fetal head 1/5 palpable per abdomen

1.31 From the list below select the five criteria which would permit an assisted vaginal delivery in an uncomplicated term pregnancy. The position of the fetal head is occipito anterior.

- ❑ A The mother has not passed urine for four hours
- ❑ B The mother does not have an epidural *in situ*
- ❑ C The head is 0/5 palpable per abdomen
- ❑ D The head is 1/5 palpable per abdomen
- ❑ E There is minimal caput and moulding
- ❑ F The station of the head is 2 cm above the spines
- ❑ G There is overlapping of the sagittal suture
- ❑ H The mother has passed urine in the last 30 minutes
- ❑ I The cervix is fully dilated
- ❑ J The mother has an epidural *in situ*

1.32 Induction of labour is at term contraindicated in

- ❑ A breech presentation
- ❑ B gestational diabetes
- ❑ C placenta praevia
- ❑ D post-maturity
- ❑ E pre-eclampsia

1.33 The two most common direct causes of maternal death in England and Wales are

- ❑ A thromboembolic disease
- ❑ B amniotic fluid embolism
- ❑ C ectopic pregnancy
- ❑ D haemorrhage
- ❑ E hypertensive disease in pregnancy

1.34 Which of the following definitions are correct?

☐ A Miscarriage is defined as the loss of a pregnancy before 28 weeks of gestation
☐ B Perinatal mortality is the total of all stillbirths and neonatal deaths in the first seven days of life per 1000 births
☐ C Maternal mortality is expressed as deaths per 100,000 births
☐ D Perinatal mortality is the total of all stillbirths and neonatal deaths in the first 28 days of life per 1000 births
☐ E Maternal mortality is expressed as deaths per 100,000 maternities

1.35 Which of the following statements are true of a neonate born at term (> 37 weeks)?

☐ A Babies born by elective Caesarean section are at increased risk of developing transient tachypnoea of the newborn
☐ B Babies born to mothers with pregnancy induced hypertension are at increased risk of needing phototherapy for neonatal jaundice
☐ C Babies born to mothers with pregnancy induced hypertension are at increased risk of developing respiratory distress syndrome
☐ D Babies born to mothers with gestational diabetes mellitus are at increased risk of developing hypoglycaemia
☐ E Babies born to mothers with pregnancy induced hypertension are at increased risk of developing hypoglycaemia

1.36 **A 75-year-old woman has been complaining of vulval irritation and itchiness for the past two years. On physical examination she has a thickened white patch of skin on the right labia majora which shows signs of ulceration. Which of the following is the most appropriate next step in the management of this patient?**

- ❏ A Prescribe an antibiotic
- ❏ B Prescribe an antifungal cream
- ❏ C Prescribe steroid cream
- ❏ D Refer to dermatology
- ❏ E Biopsy of the lesion

1.37 **A 46-year-old woman who has been happily married for 18 years complains of irregular vaginal bleeding. A transvaginal ultrasound scan suggests the presence of an endometrial polyp. Which of the following is the most appropriate management?**

- ❏ A Danazol
- ❏ B Progestogens
- ❏ C Transcervical hysteroscopic resection of the endometrium
- ❏ D Transcervical hysteroscopic polypectomy
- ❏ E Thermoablation of the endometrium

1.38 **A 25-year-old woman had her first cervical smear. The result shows mild dyskaryosis. Which of the following is the most appropriate next step in management?**

- ❏ A Repeat smear in one month
- ❏ B Repeat smear in six months
- ❏ C Repeat smear in one year
- ❏ D Colposcopy
- ❏ E Perform large loop excision of the transformation zone

1.39   Dysfunctional uterine bleeding (DUB)

❏   A   is defined as heavy irregular menstruation
❏   B   is associated with a fibroid uterus
❏   C   examination usually reveals no abnormality
❏   D   is defined as heavy regular menstruation
❏   E   indicates hysteroscopy and endometrial biopsy should
         be routinely performed in women aged less than 40

**1.40   Which of the following statements are true about
         antifibrinolytic agents in the treatment of
         menorrhagia?**

❏   A   Fibrinolytic inhibitors work by stopping thrombin
         formation in the spiral arterioles
❏   B   They decrease the blood loss by up to 80% per
         menstrual cycle
❏   C   They are most effective when taken during the menses
         only
❏   D   They can be safely used with NSAIDs
❏   E   They cannot be used long term due to their side
         effects

**1.41   Which of the following are recognised causes of
         male subfertility?**

❏   A   Klinefelter's syndrome
❏   B   Absent vas deferens
❏   C   Smoking
❏   D   Teetotalism
❏   E   Leukaemia at age 13

1.42   Endometrial ablation is indicated in

❏   A   the presence of submucosal fibroids
❏   B   the presence of endometrial hyperplasia
❏   C   dysfunctional uterine bleeding
❏   D   the presence of an endometrial polyp
❏   E   the presence of a cervical polyp

1.43 Counselling a 29-year-old woman with four children for laparoscopic sterilisation must include five of the following:

- ❏ A The operation is not available for women under the age of 30
- ❏ B The operation is irreversible
- ❏ C The operation is as effective as the Mirena IUS which is reversible
- ❏ D The operation will make the woman's periods heavier
- ❏ E The operation may not be possible laparoscopically
- ❏ F The failure rate is 1:300
- ❏ G The woman should stop taking the oral contraceptive pill four weeks before the operation
- ❏ H The failure rate is 1:600
- ❏ I The clips used may set off security alarms at airports
- ❏ J The clips used will be visible on an X-ray

1.44 A 58-year-old woman presents with a unilateral ovarian cyst accompanied by a large omental metastasis. Which of the following pre-operative blood tests should be performed?

- ❏ A LDH, βhCG, AFP
- ❏ B CEA, CA135, CA199
- ❏ C CA155, CEA, CA199
- ❏ D CA199, CEA, CA125
- ❏ E AFP, AST, βhCG

1.45 A 72-year-old woman presents with four episodes of post-menopausal bleeding over the last six months. She is otherwise fit and well although her BMI is 38 kg/m². The most likely diagnosis is

- ❏ A submucosal fibroid
- ❏ B ovarian cancer
- ❏ C endometrial cancer
- ❏ D cervical ectropion
- ❏ E vaginal cancer

1.46 The most appropriate treatment for a Bartholin's abscess is

❏ A   marsupialisation
❏ B   antibiotic therapy
❏ C   surgical excision
❏ D   incision and drainage
❏ E   observation

1.47 The most common presenting symptom of ovarian carcinoma is

❏ A   vaginal bleeding and anorexia
❏ B   weight loss and dyspareunia
❏ C   nausea and vaginal discharge
❏ D   constipation and frequent urination
❏ E   abdominal distention and pain

1.48 Cervical cancer associated with hydronephrosis would be described as which stage?

❏ A   Stage Ia
❏ B   Stage Ib
❏ C   Stage II
❏ D   Stage III
❏ E   Stage IV

1.49 Which of the following past history factors are associated with an increased risk of developing endometrial carcinoma?

❏ A   dysmenorrhoea
❏ B   dyspareunia
❏ C   endometrial polyp
❏ D   cystic hyperplasia
❏ E   dermoid cysts

1.50 **Match five of the following hormones/steroids to the statements below:**

A   Dihydroepiandrostenedione
B   Follicle stimulating hormone (FSH)
C   Gonadotrophin releasing hormone (GnRH)
D   Insulin
E   Luteinising hormone (LH)
F   Oestradiol
G   Progesterone
H   Prolactin
I   Testosterone
J   Thyroid stimulating hormone (TSH)

❏   1   is produced in a pulsatile fashion from the hypothalamus
❏   2   is increased in the postpartum period
❏   3   is produced predominantly by the thecal cells in women
❏   4   is the pituitary hormone that is stimulated by low oestradiol concentrations
❏   5   is produced predominantly by the adrenal gland in women

PAPER 1 – ANSWERS AT A GLANCE

1.1	CE	1.26	A
1.2	BCE	1.27	B
1.3	CEFHI	1.28	A
1.4	BCE	1.29	BD
1.5	AC	1.30	CE
1.6	A:4 B:8 C:9 D:6 E:1	1.31	CEHIJ
1.7	BCE	1.32	AC
1.8	BC	1.33	AE
1.9	BD	1.34	BE
1.10	ABD	1.35	AD
1.11	ACGHJ	1.36	E
1.12	ACDE	1.37	D
1.13	ACDEH	1.38	B
1.14	D	1.39	CD
1.15	C	1.40	CD
1.16	D	1.41	ABCE
1.17	D	1.42	C
1.18	B	1.43	BCEFJ
1.19	BE	1.44	D
1.20	BC	1.45	C
1.21	BEGHJ	1.46	A
1.22	BCD	1.47	E
1.23	DE	1.48	D
1.24	CE	1.49	CD
1.25	ABCDE	1.50	1:C 2:H 3:I 4:B 5:A

PAPER 1 – ANSWERS AND TEACHING NOTES

1.1   CE
The principle supports of the uterus are the transverse cervical ligaments (cardinal ligaments), uterosacral ligaments and the round ligament. The infundibular ligaments attach the ovaries to the posteo-lateral wall of the uterus. The pyriformis muscle lines the lateral wall of the pelvis overlying the iliosacral ligament.

1.2   BCE
The ovary is attached to the uterus by the infundibular ligament, the mesovarium and its blood supply which arises from the renal arteries. The pouch of Douglas is posterior to the uterus lying between the rectum and the uterus. Immediately following the LH surge the oocyte completes the first stage of meiosis extruding the first polar body which is haploid (23 chromosomes).

1.3   CEFHI
In a woman over 40 irregular vaginal bleeding may be due to any of the following; cervical ectropion, cervical polyp, cervical cancer, endometrial hyperplasia (cystic or atypical), endometrial polyp, submucosal fibroid and rarely endometrial cancer. It is unlikely that she has pelvic inflammatory disease, and chlamydia rarely causes irregular vaginal bleeding. A speculum examination is an opportunity to detect cervical abnormalities and perform a smear. A digital vaginal examination will detect an enlarged uterus suggestive of fibroids. Endometrial biopsy alone is indicated in women under 40 because the risk of malignancy is greatly reduced. A transvaginal ultrasound scan will detect endometrial polyps/submucosal fibroids and measure the endometrial thickness. A hysteroscopy and endometrial biopsy is the gold standard for detecting endometrial abnormalities in women over 40.

1.4   BCE
The urethra is only 3.5 cm long and is anterior to the lower third of the vagina. The bladder when empty lies below the uterovesical fold which arises from the junction between the uterine body and the cervix.

1.5   AC
The broad ligament is made of two layers of peritoneum that covers the fallopian tube, round ligament, and down the sides of the uterus to the cervix where anteriorly it merges into the uterovesical fold and posteriorly the peritoneum of the pouch of Douglas. The ureter, superior vesical artery and the ovarian artery are all retroperitoneal. The uterine artery is a branch of the internal iliac artery and runs between the leaves of the broad ligament along the lateral wall of the uterus.

1.6   A:4 B:8 C:9 D:6 E:1
Testosterone is produced by the thecal cells and converted to oestradiol by aromatase. Oestradiol is secreted throughout the menstrual cycle initially by the granulosa cells in the developing follicle and then by the corpus luteum. Progesterone is produced by the corpus luteum, changing the endometrium from proliferative to secretory. The LH surge triggers the final stage of the first meiotic division whilst fertilisation causes the second meiotic division with the extrusion of the polar body by uneven division of the cytoplasm. GnRH is secreted by the hypothalamus in a pulsatile manner and stimulates the production and release of LH and FSH in the anterior pituitary gland. Androgen precursors are secreted by the adrenal but oestradiol is only produced in the ovary.

1.7   BCE
Trocars placed in the iliac fossae can perforate the inferior epigastric artery while one placed centrally can perforate the bladder. The uterus can be perforated by a sound placed in the uterus to move it around.

1.8   BC
The granulosa cells produce oestradiol while the thecal cells produce the androgens androstenedione and testosterone. Prior to the LH surge the oocyte contains 46 chromosomes. The LH surge occurs at the end of the follicular phase.

1.9 BD

βhCG is produced by the developing trophoblast of the embryo. The developing trophoblastic villi of the placenta invade into the maternal capillary bed so that the endotheliums of the maternal and fetal capillaries are in close contact. The integrity of the maternal capillaries remains intact and there is no direct circulation between the maternal and fetal circulations at any time. Haemoglobin F differs from HbA by 25% of its amino acids. This allows the oxygen dissociation curve of HbF to move to the left of HbA so that for any given $p(O_2)$ concentration HbF has a greater affinity for oxygen than HbA.

1.10 ABD

The foramen ovale, the ductus arteriosus and the umbilical veins and arteries close within a few hours of birth. The breakdown of fetal blood cells in the first few days of life allows HbF to be replaced by HbA with its lower affinity for oxygen. This may lead to physiological jaundice in the newborn.

1.11 ACGHJ

βhCG is a polypeptide protein produced by the trophoblastic cells of the developing placenta. It has a half-life in plasma of 48 hours. It shares its β-subunit with luteinising hormone. It is measured using a monoclonal ELISA test. βhCG levels are raised in multiple pregnancies, Down's syndrome, hydatidiform mole, choriocarcinoma, some gonadoblastomas and dysgerminomas. In ectopic pregnancy βhCG increases at a slower rate than an ongoing intrauterine pregnancy (doubles every 48 hours).

1.12 ACDE

LH and FSH are two glycoproteins secreted by the pituitary in response to a GnRH pulse and thus have a pulsatile pattern of secretion themselves. In the middle of a 28 day cycle/at ovulation there is a sudden and large increase in the secretion of LH and FSH, the LH surge lasts for three days. LH luteinises the granulosa cells which start to produce progesterone in the corpus luteum.

1.13 ACDEH

The current average age of the menopause is 51 years. The ovaries gradually become more resistant to the action of FSH so oestrogen concentrations remain low because few or no follicles develop. This leads, by negative feedback, to an increase in FSH concentrations. LH concentrations rise later than FSH concentrations. Low oestrogen levels cause hot flushes (not FSH), and osteoporosis with loss of trabecular bone leading to vertebral crush fractures and fractures of the neck of femur. In addition atrophic vaginitis is common, often causing dyspareunia because of lack of vaginal secretions and poor elasticity of the vagina.

1.14 D

The baby can only inherit HbS from its mother but can inherit either HbA or HbS from its father. This gives a one in two chance of the baby having either sickle cell trait or sickle cell disease.

1.15 C

Amniotic fluid volume is often decreased in fetuses that are hypoxic. An increased amniotic fluid volume is associated with some congenital abnormalities while a decreased volume is found in babies with trisomy 13, 16 and 18 who often have renal agenesis. Bilirubin is only found in babies with hydropic disease of the newborn, most commonly due to rhesus isoimmunisation.

1.16 D

Sickle cell disease and cystic fibrosis are autosomal recessive whilst Duchenne muscular dystrophy and haemophilia are X-linked recessive disorders.

1.17 D

Skene's glands are associated with the urethra. The uterine wall does not produce secretions. The endocervical glands and Bartholin's glands are insignificant contributors to vaginal lubrication.

1.18 B
Mastitis, wound infections or haematomas will give a pyrexia but are not associated with prolonged vaginal bleeding. It is rare for products of conception to be found following a Caesarean section since the cavity is checked at the time of operation. Endometritis is however common following Caesarean section.

1.19 BE
Escherichia coli is a normal gastrointestinal commensal. *Staphylococcus aureus* is a normal commensal of skin and if found in the vagina can cause toxic shock syndrome. *Candida albicans* is a yeast which causes thrush.

1.20 BC
Vaginal examination at a routine antenatal visit is unnecessary and uncomfortable. Cardiotocography is indicated if there is any concern about fetal well-being, eg if the mother reports reduced fetal movements. Haemoglobin is checked at booking, 26–28 and 32–34 weeks. Urinalysis and listening to the fetal heart with a handheld Doppler device or Pinard's stethoscope are performed at each antenatal visit.

1.21 BEGHJ
GDM is the onset of diabetes in pregnancy and usually arises beyond 28 weeks. Women who are at risk of developing GDM include those with a first degree relative with type 2 diabetes (not type 1). Persistent glucose levels over 8 mmol/l increases the chances of the baby becoming macrosomic (fetal abdominal circumference > 90th centile) and of intrauterine death beyond 40 weeks. The renal threshold for releasing glucose into the urine is lower in pregnancy and so it is more common for the urine to be positive for glucose in pregnancy. Women with type 1 diabetes prior to pregnancy have a three fold increased risk of congenital abnormality if their diabetes is poorly controlled.

1.22   BCD
Danazol may masculinise a female fetus. Women on warfarin should be changed to heparin during the first trimester of pregnancy while organogenesis is occurring. All anti-epileptic drugs are teratogenic. However, sodium valproate is the least teratogenic and the risk of an epileptic fit to the fetus and the mother outweighs the teratogenic risk. The teratogenicity of ACE inhibitors has not been fully established so they are not used in pregnancy in case they have a teratogenic potential.

1.23   DE
Pregnancy induced hypertension without proteinuria most commonly arises at term. It can be safely treated with methyldopa while awaiting spontaneous labour. The fetus is usually normally grown; there is no excess risk of intrauterine death or cephalo-pelvic disproportion.

1.24   CE
The early signs of pregnancy include breast tenderness, secondary amenorrhoea, urinary frequency and nausea. Varicose veins may arise de novo or become symptomatic in pregnancy but they are not typical of early pregnancy.

1.25   ABCDE
Due to limited resources, routine fetal echocardiography is not offered to all women. High risk patients such as those included above in addition to other maternal diseases (connective tissue disorder, phenylketonuria, rubella, parvovirus and Coxsackie virus), detection of another anomaly, raised nuchal thickness, fetal arrhythmia, hydrops and polyhydramnios should be referred for fetal echocardiography.

1.26   A
A significantly raised MSAFP is most likely to indicate a neural tube defect. Ventral wall defects are much less common than NTDs. A dating scan at 11 weeks is one of the most accurate ways of determining gestation so it is highly unlikely that the raised level is secondary to 'wrong dates'. Bleeding in pregnancy is not associated with a raised MSAFP. MSAFP usually falls following the demise of the fetus.

1.27 B

At 28 weeks around 10% of babies are presenting by the breech. By term (37 completed weeks of pregnancy) only 3% are still breech. Only a few babies will spontaneously turn after 37 weeks, so external cephalic version should be offered between 37 and 39 weeks.

1.28 A

The first stage of labour is divided into two phases, the latent phase and the active phase. The latent phase involves effacement (shortening and thinning) and dilatation of the cervix to 3 cm. The active phase involves the dilatation of the cervix from 3 cm to 10 cm. The transitional phase is used to describe the last stages of the active phase as the cervix becomes fully dilated. The second stage of labour is from full dilatation to the delivery of the baby and the third stage is the delivery of the placenta.

1.29 BD

The chances of a successful vaginal birth following a Caesarean section for a non-recurrent cause are 70%. The risk of wound dehiscence is 1–2%.

1.30 CE

In a woman who has an epidural, standard practice is to wait one hour after full dilation before starting the active phase of the second stage (pushing). Decisions regarding mode of delivery are usually made after one hour (two hours after full dilation). In situation A the head may rotate to occipito-anterior with pushing and thus achieve a normal vaginal delivery. Assisted vaginal delivery is contraindicated if the fetal head is palpable per abdomen since it increases the risk of fetal and maternal birth trauma.

1.31 CEHIJ

The criteria for attempting a vaginal delivery include full engagement of the head (0/5 palpable per abdomen, below the spines vaginally). The cervix should be fully dilated, there should be no signs of obstruction (overlapping sagittal suture is a sign of outlet obstruction), the mother should have an empty bladder (emptied within last 30 minutes or catheterised), and there should be adequate analgesia (epidural or pudendal block).

1.32 AC
Induction of labour is contraindicated in breech presentations at term because of the risk of entrapment of the after coming head. In placenta praevia cervical dilatation will cause bleeding by shearing off the placental bed. Induction of labour is routinely offered to women who are more than ten days beyond their expected date of delivery (post maturity) or at 40 weeks for women with GDM because of the small increased risk of intrauterine death. Induction of labour is offered to women with PET at term in order to reduce the risk of eclampsia.

1.33 AE
In the last two triennia thromboembolic disease and hypertensive disease of pregnancy have been the two commonest causes of maternal death. The others listed are all important causes of maternal death, with haemorrhage and amniotic fluid embolism a close third and fourth.

1.34 BE
Miscarriage is defined as the loss of a pregnancy before 24 weeks of gestation. The definition was changed in 1994 following changes to the Abortion Act. Maternal mortality is expressed either as deaths per 1000 births or 100,000 maternities.

1.35 AD
Babies born to mothers with pregnancy induced hypertension do not have an increased risk of problems in the neonatal period.

1.36 E
The most likely diagnosis is that this woman has lichen sclerosus. The ulcerated area may be malignant and so an urgent vulval biopsy is indicated.

1.37 D
There is no indication for ablation of the whole endometrium in this woman. Danazol and progestogens are used to treat endometrial hyperplasia.

1.38   B

Mild dyskaryosis can revert to normal in young women after six months and therefore a repeat smear should be performed after six months. Colposcopy is indicated if the second smear is positive. Loop excision is rarely indicated in mild dyskaryosis, the majority can be successfully treated with cold coagulation.

1.39   CD

DUB is defined as heavy, regular menstruation without any pathological cause detected (on history, examination or investigation). Fibroids are a pathological cause of menorrhagia and are often associated with heavy regular menstruation. Hysteroscopy and endometrial biopsy are only indicated in women over the age of 40 or if an abnormality is detected on transvaginal ultrasound scan.

1.40   CD

Antifibrinolytic agents work by stopping fibrinolysis of the clots in the spiral arterioles. This is effective in 50% of cases and decreases the menstrual loss by up to 40% in women proven to have heavy periods. They have a limited number of minor side effects, can be safely taken with NSAIDs and are taken only during menstruation.

1.41   ABCE

Klinefelter's syndrome carries the karyotype XXY and is associated with azoospermia or severe oligospermia. Absent vas deferens does not allow the sperm to leave the testicle and leads to azoospermia. Smoking and drinking both affect spermatogenesis. Chemotherapy for leukaemia at puberty is associated with male subfertility.

1.42   C

Endometrial ablation is only indicated if no pathological cause for menorrhagia has been found.

1.43   BCEFJ
In addition, the discussion should include other forms of contraception including vasectomy for her partner. The stability of the relationship should also be explored because she is below the age of 30. There is no indication for the woman to stop the OCP as the operation is performed as a day case, and she will mobilise within hours. Stopping the OCP increases the risk of failure of the operation as the woman may have already conceived at the time of the operation even if the pregnancy test is negative. A pregnancy test should always be performed on the day of the operation. The three essential facts that the woman must be told and recorded in the notes are the risk of failure (1:300), that the procedure is permanent and irreversible, and that she may require a mini-laparotomy. The remainder are best practice.

1.44   D
These are the tumour markers for epithelial ovarian cancer which is the commonest form of ovarian cancer in older women. Those listed in A are tumour markers for germ cell tumours which are more common in younger women.

1.45   C
Submucosal fibroids become quiescent following the menopause and usually calcify. There is no evidence of increased risk of endometrial cancer in women with fibroids. Ovarian cancer rarely if ever presents with postmenopausal bleeding. Cervical ectropion is a condition of young women. Vaginal cancer is very rare and usually presents with vaginal discharge.

1.46   A
Antibiotic therapy usually gives some relief but the abscess recurs shortly afterwards. Excision can cause scarring and pain and is reserved for recurrent abscesses. The eversion of the edges at marsupialisation prevents the abscess from resealing and recurring.

1.47   E
Ovarian carcinoma rarely causes significant symptoms until its later stages, which explains the late presentation of these women.

1.48 D
Stages Ia and Ib refer to tumour confined to the cervix, stage II is spread into the parametrium or beyond the upper third of the vagina, stage III is spread outside the pelvis but within the abdomen and stage IV is spread beyond the abdominal cavity. Hydonephrosis in cervical carcinoma is most commonly caused by the expansion of the tumour to the pelvic side-walls causing obstruction of the ureter. Since the ureter is retroperitoneal and its obstruction causes renal pelvis dilatation this is considered extension beyond the pelvis.

1.49 CD
Endometrial carcinoma is associated with unopposed oestrogen whose early manifestations include endometrial polyps, cystic hyperplasia and atypical endometrial hyperplasia.

1.50   1:C 2:H 3:I 4:B 5:A
GnRH is released in a pulsatile fashion from the hypothalamus and acts on the pituitary to increase FSH and LH secretion from the pituitary. Low concentrations of oestradiol have a direct stimulating effect on FSH but not LH. Prolactin is raised in the postpartum period so that lactation can occur. TSH levels remain normal in pregnancy although thyroid binding globulin rises. In women dihydroepiandrostenedione is a steroid produced predominantly by the adrenal gland while testosterone is produced by the thecal cells in the ovary. Oestradiol is produced by aromatisation of testosterone in the granulosa cells and progesterone is produced by the granulosa cells after exposure to LH.

PRACTICE PAPER 2

PRACTICE PAPER 2

2.1   The ovary

☐ A   lies inferior to the fallopian tube
☐ B   is covered by the broad ligament
☐ C   has an outer medulla and an inner cortex
☐ D   contains approximately 500,000 primordial oocytes at
        menarche
☐ E   granulosa cells produce androgens

**2.2   Which of the following statements are true about
        the blood supply to the ovary?**

☐ A   It only comes through the ovarian artery
☐ B   The ovarian artery is a branch of the internal iliac
        artery
☐ C   The left ovarian vein drains into the left renal vein
☐ D   The right ovarian vein drains into the right renal vein
☐ E   The ovaries are mainly supplied by direct branches
        from the aorta

**2.3   Which of the following are absolute contra-
        indications to the insertion of an intrauterine
        contraceptive device (IUCD)?**

☐ A   A history of pelvic inflammatory disease four years ago
☐ B   Previous pregnancy with an IUCD four years ago
☐ C   Abnormal genital bleeding
☐ D   Nulliparity
☐ E   History of post-partum endometritis four years ago

2.4   The cervix

☐ A   consists mostly of smooth muscle
☐ B   consists mostly of connective tissue
☐ C   canal is lined by squamous cell epithelium
☐ D   canal is lined by cuboidal epithelium
☐ E   canal is lined by columnar epithelium

2.5   Which of the following are branches of the internal iliac artery?

❏ A   Inferior epigastric artery
❏ B   Uterine artery
❏ C   Ovarian artery
❏ D   Internal pudendal artery
❏ E   Inferior mesenteric artery

2.6   Which of the following statements are true concerning the fallopian tube?

❏ A   At ovulation there is a reversal of peristalsis
❏ B   The ampulla is the commonest site within the fallopian tube for fertilisation to take place
❏ C   Oestrogen increases peristalsis of the fallopian tube
❏ D   The fallopian tube produces nutrients for the developing embryo
❏ E   The fimbriae are essential for collection of the mature oocyte

2.7   In pregnancy

❏ A   maternal cardiac output increases by 20% compared to the non-pregnant state
❏ B   blood pressure tends to rise in the second trimester
❏ C   the main increase in circulating volume is secondary to an increase in red blood cell numbers
❏ D   respiratory rate rises secondary to increased progesterone concentrations
❏ E   there is hypermotility of the alimentary tract

2.8 **Match the following A–E to five of the statements below:**

A Progesterone
B The number of placental lobules is fixed by
C The genital organs are differentiated by
D The placenta
E Human placental lactogen

☐ 1 12 weeks from LMP
☐ 2 metabolism relaxes the uterine muscle
☐ 3 14 weeks from LMP
☐ 4 alters glucose and insulin
☐ 5 six weeks from LMP
☐ 6 grows by proliferation
☐ 7 is produced by thecal cells
☐ 8 is inhibited by LH
☐ 9 is sampled in amniocentesis
☐ 10 eight weeks from LMP

2.9 **Choose from the following statements five best matched about ovulation**

☐ A In a 30 day menstrual cycle ovulation occurs on the 10th day
☐ B The duration of the follicular phase is constant
☐ C Occurs when the follicle reaches a diameter of 12–14 mm
☐ D The duration of the luteal phase is constant
☐ E Occurs when the oestradiol levels are usually greater than 800 pmol/l
☐ F Ovulation occurs on the 16th day when cycle is of 30 days
☐ G Usually ovulation occurs from the same ovary each month
☐ H The duration of a normal follicular phase is from 12–14 days
☐ I Occurs when the follicular diameter reaches 18–25 mm
☐ J The granulosa cells start producing progesterone

2.10 Progestogen level is high in

❏ A the follicular phase of the menstrual cycle
❏ B pregnancy
❏ C choriocarcinoma
❏ D ectopic pregnancy
❏ E the luteal phase of the menstrual cycle

2.11 The corpus luteum

❏ A secretes only progesterone
❏ B secretes both oestrogen and progesterone
❏ C degeneration leads to the onset of menstruation
❏ D is necessary for pregnancy continuation
❏ E is a benign ovarian cyst

2.12 Choose from the following five statements best matched about the endometrium

❏ A Progesterone is important for the normal development of the endometrium
❏ B Oestrogen is not important for normal endometrial growth
❏ C Abnormal menstruation may be caused by abnormalities of endometrial growth
❏ D Prolonged exposure to oestrogen predisposes the endometrium to malignant change
❏ E Regeneration of the endometrium is controlled by progesterone
❏ F Spasm of the arterioles is under the control of prostaglandins
❏ G Prostaglandins prevent the onset of menstruation
❏ H Spasm of the arterioles is under the control of progesterone in the endometrium
❏ I Excessive fibrinolysis may lead to breakdown of the clots that close the arterioles resulting in heavy bleeding
❏ J The average blood loss at menstruation is 90 ml

2.13   Which one of the following statements is true of cervical intraepithelial neoplasia 3 (CIN 3)?

❑   A   It can be accurately diagnosed from a cervical smear
❑   B   Abnormal cells are found throughout the epidermis of the cervical skin
❑   C   It is caused by HIV
❑   D   Women with CIN 3 who are not treated rarely develop invasive cervical cancer
❑   E   It is often found in women who are virgo intacta

2.14   Which of the following statements are true of maternal changes in pregnancy?

❑   A   Cardiac output increases by 20% in the first trimester
❑   B   Respiratory rate increases secondary to the effects of oestradiol
❑   C   Cardiac output increases by 40% in the first trimester
❑   D   Renal plasma flow increases by 10–20%
❑   E   Renal plasma flow increases by 30–50%

2.15   Which of the following disorders is inherited as an autosomal recessive disorder?

❑   A   Cystic fibrosis
❑   B   Huntington's chorea
❑   C   Androgen insensitivity syndrome
❑   D   von Willibrand's disease
❑   E   Hurler's syndrome

2.16   Which of the following are recognised as causing the changes in the ECG during pregnancy?

❑   A   The diaphragm pushes the heart upwards into the chest
❑   B   The left ventricular volume decreases
❑   C   The aorta dilates
❑   D   The left ventricular volume increases
❑   E   The aortic arch unfolds

2.17 Concerning endometrial carcinoma

❏ A at stage 1 the carcinoma has penetrated into one third of the myometrium
❏ B the prognosis is worse if the surrounding endometrium is normal
❏ C it commonly presents with post-coital bleeding
❏ D it is commonly a squamous cell carcinoma
❏ E it is commonly an adenocarcinoma

2.18 Match five of the following hormones/steroids to the statements below:

A Antidiuretic hormone
B Cortisol
C Dihydroepiandrostenedione
D Gonadotrophin releasing hormone (GnRH)
E Insulin
F Oestradiol
G Oxytocin
H Progesterone
I Prolactin
J Prostglandin E2

❏ 1 is thought to be produced by the fetus as a trigger for the onset of labour
❏ 2 is increased by nipple stimulation
❏ 3 a decrease in production occurs just prior to the onset of labour
❏ 4 is inhibited by dopamine
❏ 5 is associated with a change in the collagen matrix of the cervix

2.19 Abnormalities in a fetus can be caused by

❏ A varicella
❏ B herpes simplex virus 2
❏ C parvovirus
❏ D human papilloma virus
❏ E human immunodeficiency virus

2.20 In the majority of cases the 20 week fetal anomaly ultrasound scan should detect

❏ A   duodenal atresia
❏ B   tracheoesophageal fistula
❏ C   exomphalos
❏ D   renal agenesis
❏ E   Fallot's tetralogy

2.21 Abdominal pain in pregnancy may be caused by

❏ A   appendicitis
❏ B   constipation
❏ C   breech presentation
❏ D   urinary tract infection
❏ E   placental abruption

2.22 Which five of the following ten statements are true?

❏ A   Pre-eclampsia is defined as a rise in diastolic blood pressure of > 15 mmHg from the blood pressure at less than twelve weeks with proteinuria of > 300 mg/ 24 h
❏ B   Blood pressure should be stabilised before induction of labour
❏ C   Women with pre-eclampsia should be delivered by Caesarean section
❏ D   Women with pre-eclampsia may develop epigastric pain
❏ E   Women with pre-eclampsia are at lower risk of developing a deep vein thrombosis
❏ F   In the majority of cases pre-eclampsia develops before 32 weeks gestation
❏ G   Pre-eclampsia increases the risk of a placental abruption
❏ H   Magnesium sulphate is the treatment of choice for lowering blood pressure
❏ I   Women with pre-eclampsia may develop oliguria
❏ J   Pretibial oedema is diagnostic of pre-eclampsia

2.23 Concerning anaemia in pregnancy which of the following are true?

❏ A Women with a haemoglobin of less than 10.5 g/dl should be given iron supplements

❏ B It may be associated with a haemoglobinopathy

❏ C The majority of pregnant women have a physiological reduction in haemoglobin concentration

❏ D Vitamin B_{12} deficiency is common in pregnancy

❏ E Women with a haemoglobin of less than 10 g/dl at 40 weeks gestation should be given a 2 unit transfusion

2.24 Which one of the following statements is false?

❏ A Smoking cessation in pregnancy reduces the risk of premature labour

❏ B Abstinence from sexual intercourse reduces the risk of antepartum haemorrhage in women with placenta praevia

❏ C Strict bed rest reduces the risk of first trimester miscarriage

❏ D Eating unpasteurized cheese increases the risk of the baby developing listeriosis

❏ E Excess alcohol intake during pregnancy increases the risk of delivering a small for gestational age baby

2.25 Which one of the following statements about CNS/neural tube defect anomaly is true?

❏ A Ultrasound scanning detects 70% of fetuses with anencephaly

❏ B Ultrasound scanning detects 42% spina bifida

❏ C The level of the defect in spina bifida has no prognostic predictive value

❏ D Spina bifida at L4/L5 is incompatible with survival beyond one year of age

❏ E Pre-conceptual folic acid significantly reduces the risk of neural tube defect

2.26 **A 25-year-old woman in her first pregnancy presents at 26 weeks of gestation with a small amount of vaginal bleeding. An ultrasound at 20 weeks reported that the placenta was posterior and fundal. Her blood group is A Rh negative. Which of the following is the most appropriate treatment?**

- ❏ A 500 mg Erythromycin
- ❏ B 2 units Blood transfusion
- ❏ C 500 IU Anti D
- ❏ D 10 units Erythropoietin
- ❏ E 500 mg Ethambutal

2.27 **A 22-year-old woman in her first pregnancy presents to labour ward at 32 weeks gestation. She is complaining of severe abdominal pain and vaginal bleeding. Which of the following is the most likely diagnosis?**

- ❏ A Placenta praevia
- ❏ B Placenta accreta
- ❏ C Placenta increta
- ❏ D Placenta percreta
- ❏ E Placenta abruption

2.28 **A 22-year-old woman in her first pregnancy presents to labour ward at 32 weeks gestation. She is complaining of severe abdominal pain and vaginal bleeding. Which of the following are appropriate for the immediate management of this woman?**

- ❏ A Group and save
- ❏ B Cardiotocography
- ❏ C Central venous pressure line (CVP)
- ❏ D 500 ml normal saline
- ❏ E Full blood count

2.29 The Bishop's score is used to assess

❏ A   the pelvic diameters
❏ B   the recommended method of delivery antenatally
❏ C   the recommended method of induction of labour
❏ D   the recommended method of delivery in labour
❏ E   the presentation of the fetus

2.30 Breech presentation of a chromosomally normal fetus

❏ A   occurs in 2–3% of pregnancies at term
❏ B   is associated with fetal congenital dislocation of the hips
❏ C   is associated with fetal neural tube defects
❏ D   is associated with fetal cardiac anomalies
❏ E   occurs in 10% of pregnancies at term

2.31 Which of the following statements are true for pregnant women who are human immunodeficiency virus positive?

❏ A   Antiretroviral agents taken during pregnancy increase the risk of fetal abnormality
❏ B   Antiretroviral agents taken during pregnancy reduce the risk of vertical transmission from 45% to 23%
❏ C   Breast feeding should be encouraged
❏ D   Breast feeding should be discouraged
❏ E   Antiretroviral agents taken during pregnancy reduce the risk of vertical transmission from 25% to 8%

2.32 Which of the following statements are true with regard to a right medio-lateral (RML) episiotomy?

❏ A A RML episiotomy reduces the risk of a third degree tear

❏ B An episiotomy should be performed if there is evidence of shoulder dystocia

❏ C An episiotomy should be performed as the head is crowning if there is evidence of fetal distress

❏ D An episiotomy is indicated in all assisted vaginal deliveries

❏ E An episiotomy should be performed if there is evidence that the woman is going to sustain a perineal tear

2.33 A woman presents at 34 weeks gestation complaining of itching. Her pregnancy is otherwise uncomplicated. What is the most appropriate action to take?

❏ A Refer her to a dermatologist

❏ B Give her two intramuscular steroid injections 12 hours apart

❏ C Give her a topical steroid cream

❏ D Check her liver function tests

❏ E Check her renal function and urate levels

2.34 Breast feeding has been shown to

❏ A increase the risk of the mother developing breast cancer

❏ B reduce the risk of the mother developing ovarian cancer

❏ C reduce the risk of the mother developing breast cancer

❏ D reduce the risk of gastrointestinal infections in the baby

❏ E reduce the risk of viral infections in the early weeks of life

2.35 **The risk of premature delivery is increased by**

☐ A   urinary tract infection
☐ B   obesity
☐ C   essential hypertension
☐ D   smoking
☐ E   anorexia

2.36 **A 22-year-old woman presents with mouth ulcer, sore throat, vaginal discharge, fever and myalgia. She has a temperature of 38.3°C, cervical and inguinal lymphadenopathy, exudative pharyngitis and multiple ulcers on the oral mucosa, the labia and cervix. Which of the following is the most likely diagnosis?**

☐ A   *Trichomonas vaginalis*
☐ B   Gonorrhoea
☐ C   Herpes simplex virus
☐ D   Candidiasis
☐ E   Syphilis

2.37 **A 64-year-old woman comes to the GP complaining of 'leaking' urine. She describes these episodes as small squirts of urine that come out whenever she laughs, coughs, sneezes or engages in physical activity. Urine culture is negative. Urodynamic test performed is normal. Which of the following is the most likely diagnosis?**

☐ A   Detrusor instability (DI)
☐ B   Genuine stress urinary incontinence (GSUI)
☐ C   Neurogenic bladder
☐ D   Pyelonephritis
☐ E   Urinary tract infection

2.38 **Benign teratomas (dermoid cysts)**

☐ A   are bilateral in 10% of women with a benign teratoma
☐ B   commonly present with secondary amenorrhoea
☐ C   can be diagnosed on plain abdominal X-ray
☐ D   are very rare in women aged under 25
☐ E   are associated with an increased risk of cyst rupture

2.39 **A 26-year-old woman attends the Early Pregnancy Assessment Unit at seven weeks with lower abdominal pain. A transvaginal ultrasound scan confirms an ongoing seven-week intrauterine pregnancy with 4 x 4 cm right ovarian simple cyst. Which of the following is the most appropriate next step in the management of this cyst?**

- ❏ A Urgent ovarian cystectomy
- ❏ B Aspiration of the cyst
- ❏ C Laparoscopy
- ❏ D Reassure that it is a normal finding
- ❏ E Termination of the pregnancy

2.40 **Concerning menorrhagia**

- ❏ A blood loss exceeds 80 ml per menstrual cycle
- ❏ B female sterilisation is a recognised cause of menorrhagia
- ❏ C thyroid disease is a recognised cause of menorrhagia
- ❏ D systemic coagulation disorders are a recognised cause of menorrhagia
- ❏ E blood loss exceeds 60 ml per menstrual cycle

2.41 **The commonest cause of anovulatory subfertility is**

- ❏ A Turner's syndrome
- ❏ B hyperprolactinaemia
- ❏ C polycystic ovary syndrome
- ❏ D hypogonadotrophic hypogonadism
- ❏ E Asherman's syndrome

2.42 **Endometriosis**

- ❏ A is a condition that causes constant abdominal pain
- ❏ B is a condition that causes cyclical abdominal pain
- ❏ C is a cause of dyspareurnia
- ❏ D is a common cause of tubal infertility
- ❏ E is a condition that causes anovulation

2.43 **A 19-year-old woman presents to the Accident and Emergency department with severe lower abdominal pain. Her last menstrual period was ten days ago. Select the most likely diagnosis from the list A–J for each of the scenarios described below**

A   Appendicitis
B   Bleeding into a right ovarian cyst
C   Diverticulitis
D   Ectopic pregnancy
E   Endometriosis
F   Inevitable miscarriage
G   Pelvic inflammatory disease
H   Rupture of a right ovarian cyst
I   Small bowel obstruction
J   Torsion of a right ovarian cyst

❏   1   Her lower abdomen is tender on the right with cervical excitation. She has no nausea or vomiting. There is a suggestion of a right adnexal mass. Her pregnancy test is negative.

❏   2   Her lower abdomen is tender on the right with cervical excitation. She has some nausea but no vomiting. There is a suggestion of a right adnexal mass. Her pregnancy test is positive.

❏   3   Her lower abdomen is tender on the right with cervical excitation. She has nausea and vomiting. There is a suggestion of a right adnexal mass. Her pregnancy test is negative.

❏   4   Her lower abdomen is tender on the right with no cervical excitation. She has nausea and vomiting. Her temperature is 37.6°C. Her pregnancy test is negative.

❏   5   Her lower abdomen is tender bilaterally with bilateral cervical excitation. She has nausea but no vomiting. Her temperature is 38.6°C. Her pregnancy test is negative.

2.44 **A 58-year-old woman presents with a unilateral ovarian cyst accompanied by a large omental metastasis. The most appropriate post-operative treatment is**

❏ A cisplatin alone
❏ B carboplatin and taxol
❏ C bleomycin, cisplatin and etoposide
❏ D taxol alone
❏ E carboplatin alone

2.45 **Which of the following statements are true about cervical squamocarcinoma?**

❏ A It is associated with human papilloma virus
❏ B Stage I disease is treated with intracavity radiotherapy
❏ C The primary treatment for stage III disease is chemotherapy
❏ D The primary treatment for stage III disease is radiotherapy
❏ E It is associated with herpes simplex virus

2.46 **The most effective chemotherapeutic agent in the management of recurrent endometrial carcinoma is**

❏ A antimetabolites
❏ B progestogens
❏ C alkylating agents
❏ D vinca alkaloids
❏ E carboplatin

2.47 **In which of the following scenarios is surgery indicated for an adnexal mass?**

❏ A A 5 cm cyst in a 23-year-old with pelvic inflammatory disease
❏ B A 5 cm cyst in a 53-year-old which has echogenic foci
❏ C A 5 cm cyst in a 23-year-old who is 10 weeks pregnant
❏ D A 5 cm cyst in a 23-year-old which has echogenic foci
❏ E A 5 cm cyst in a 23-year-old which is described as haemorrhagic

2.48 **Long-term complications of vaginal hysterectomy and antero-posterior repair include**

❑ A rectal mucosal prolapse
❑ B diverticulitis
❑ C urinary retention
❑ D enterocele
❑ E vaginal vault prolapse

2.49 **The legal reasons for performing termination of pregnancy include:**

❑ A The fetus is less than 24 weeks and continuation of the pregnancy would endanger the physical or mental health of the mother greater than if the pregnancy was terminated.
❑ B The fetus is greater than 24 weeks and continuation of the pregnancy would endanger the physical or mental health of the mother greater than if the pregnancy was terminated.
❑ C The fetus is less than 24 weeks and continuation of the pregnancy would endanger the financial health of the mother greater than if the pregnancy was terminated.
❑ D The fetus is greater than 24 weeks and has abnormalities that pose a significant risk that the child will suffer from significant disability.
❑ E The fetus is less than 24 weeks and the mother's situation is not compatible with continuing with the pregnancy.

2.50 **A woman of 72 presents with four episodes of post-menopausal bleeding over the last six months. An endometrial biopsy is reported as well-differentiated adeno-carcinoma. An MRI scan shows no evidence of spread. She is otherwise fit and well although her BMI is 38 kg/m². The most appropriate treatment is**

- ❏ A provera
- ❏ B transcervical resection of the endometrium
- ❏ C total abdominal hysterectomy
- ❏ D total abdominal hysterectomy and bilateral salpingo-oophorectomy
- ❏ E Wertheim's hysterectomy

PAPER 2 – ANSWERS AT A GLANCE

2.1	AD	2.26	C
2.2	CE	2.27	E
2.3	AC	2.28	BE
2.4	BE	2.29	C
2.5	BD	2.30	ABC
2.6	ABDE	2.31	DE
2.7	D	2.32	BC
2.8	A:2 B:1 C:10 D:6 E:4	2.33	D
2.9	DEFIJ	2.34	CDE
2.10	BCE	2.35	ACDE
2.11	BCDE	2.36	C
2.12	ACDFI	2.37	B
2.13	B	2.38	AC
2.14	CE	2.39	D
2.15	A	2.40	ACD
2.16	ADE	2.41	C
2.17	BE	2.42	BC
2.18	1:B 2:G 3:H 4:I 5:J	2.43	1:B 2:D 3:J 4:A 5:G
2.19	AC	2.44	B
2.20	ACD	2.45	AD
2.21	ABDE	2.46	B
2.22	ABDGI	2.47	BD
2.23	ABC	2.48	DE
2.24	C	2.49	AD
2.25	E	2.50	D

PAPER 2 – ANSWERS AND TEACHING NOTES

2.1 AD
The ovary has an outer cortex and an inner medulla. It is attached to the back of the broad ligament by a fold of peritoneum called the mesovarium which carries part of the blood supply, lymphatic drainage and nerve supply. The granulosa cells secrete oestradiol converted from the androgens produced by the thecal cells.

2.2 CE
The main arterial supply to the ovaries arises from the aorta, just above the inferior mesenteric artery although the exact site varies from individual to individual. The ovary is supplied by the ovarian artery and arcuate artery arising from the uterine artery. The venous drainage on the right is directly into the inferior vena cava but on the left is into the left renal vein.

2.3 AC
A past history of PID increases the risk of future episodes and the IUCD is associated with an increased risk of PID. A previous pregnancy with an IUCD is not a contraindication but it is unlikely that a woman who has fallen pregnant while using an IUCD will accept it as a reliable form of contraception. Following endometritis after pregnancy there is no increased risk with an IUCD provided the infection has been adequately treated.

2.4 BE
Smooth muscle is found round the internal and external os which act like sphincters. In the non-pregnant state the cervix consists mostly of connective tissue (collagen). In late pregnancy the matrix of the connective tissue becomes softer with a greater water content. The cervical canal is lined by columnar epithelium, the external surface of the cervix is covered by squamous epithelium.

2.5 BD
The inferior epigastric artery is a branch of the external iliac artery. The inferior mesenteric artery and the ovarian artery are branches from the aorta.

2.6   ABDE
Oestrogen reduces the motility of the tube. The fallopian tube has four parts going from the uterus to the ovary – the intramural (cornual), isthmus, ampulla, infundibulum which ends with the fimbriae.

2.7   D
Maternal cardiac output rises by 40% during pregnancy. The increased circulating volume is due to an increase in plasma volume. The number of red cells does increase but the effect is diluted so that women who are pregnant have lower haemoglobin concentrations than in the non-pregnant state despite the greater number of circulating red cells. Progesterone increases respiratory rate and decreases motility in the gastrointestinal tract.

2.8   A:2 B:1 C:10 D:6 E:4
Progesterone relaxes the myometrium and exerts a negative feedback on LH. Testosterone and androstenedione are produced by thecal cells. The placenta is sampled in chorionic villous sampling and the amniotic fluid at amniocentesis.

2.9   DEFIJ
The normal duration of the follicular phase is between 9 and 18 days while the luteal phase is more constant at 12–14 days, therefore ovulation is usually assumed to occur 14 days prior to the next period (30 – 14 = 16). Ovulation usually occurs at oestradiol levels of 800–1200 pmol/l and a follicular diameter of 18–25 mm. The high levels of oestradiol trigger the LH surge which luteinises the granulosa cells to start producing progesterone as well as oestradiol. Ovulation may occur in either ovary and commonly alternates.

2.10   BCE
Progesterone levels rise in the luteal phase of the menstrual cycle. In pregnancy the corpus luteum is maintained by the action of βhCG so progesterone levels remain high and rise in the early stages of pregnancy. In abnormal pregnancies the progesterone levels tend to be low and this can be of diagnostic assistance in ectopic pregnancy and miscarriage. Chorio-carcinoma is associated with raised levels of hCG and so progesterone levels are often high.

2.11 BCDE
After the follicle ruptures it changes to become the corpus luteum, which secretes progesterone under the stimulation of LH. If pregnancy does not result then the corpus luteum starts to degenerate. This withdraws hormonal support from the endometrium and menstruation begins.

2.12 ACDFI
Oestrogen and progesterone are both essential in the normal development of the endometrium and initiation of menstruation. Abnormal oestrogen and progesterone levels and their timing during the menstrual cycle may lead to abnormal endometrial growth and abnormal menstruation. Spasm of the arterioles appears to be under the control of prostaglandins in the endometrium. Local clotting mechanisms are important for menstrual flow. Fibrinolysis leads to the breakdown of clots which normally close the arterioles. Menstrual loss is also dependent on the speed of endometrial regeneration which is dependent on oestrogen. Prolonged exposure of the endometrium to unopposed oestrogen increases the risk of developing endometrial hyperplasia leading eventually to endometrial carcinoma. Ovulation leads to the normal development of the endometrium and normal menstruation. The average menstrual loss is 30 ml with a range of 15–180 ml.

2.13 B
The relationship between the dysplasia seen on a cervical smear and the grade of cervical intraepithelial neoplasm is not absolute which is why women with an abnormal smear are referred to colposcopy clinics for further examination and a cervical biopsy or loop excision of the transformation zone. In CIN 1 a proportion of women will revert to having normal cervical cells with no treatment whilst those with CIN 3 commonly go on to develop cervical cancer. CIN is associated with certain forms of the human papilloma virus which is sexually transmitted and so CIN and cervical cancer are very rare in women who are virgo intacta.

2.14 CE
The respiratory rate increases because of the effect of progesterone.

2.15   A
Huntington's chorea and Hurler's syndrome are autosomal dominant. Androgen insensitivity syndrome is due to a deletion in the androgen receptor gene on the X chromosome. von Willibrand's disease is a variation of haemophilia (reduced factor 9) and is usually X-linked.

2.16   ADE
As the uterus grows the diaphragm is unable to descend during inspiration. The increased total circulating blood volume increases left ventricular volume. Changes in the collagen of the aorta and the position of the heart unfolds the aortic arch.

2.17   BE
Stage 1 disease is carcinoma confined to the endometrium with no invasion into the myometrium. It usually presents with post-menopausal bleeding. Squamous cell carcinoma is more common in cervical cancer.

2.18   1:B 2:G 3:H 4:I 5:J
There are many factors that are thought to precipitate the onset of labour. These include a drop in progesterone and relaxin, release of cortisol from the fetal adrenals, an increase in prostaglandin production by the placenta and release of oxytocin by the maternal pituitary. Stimulation of the nipples release oxytocin from the pituitary and is called the let-down reflex during lactation. Bromocriptine is a dopamine agonist used for treating hyperprolactinaemia to inhibit prolactin production.

2.19   AC
Herpes simplex virus 2 causes genital herpes. Human papilloma virus is associated with an increased risk of developing cervical cancer. Human immunodeficiency virus is associated with an increased risk of intrauterine death of an otherwise normal baby.

2.20 ACD

Duodenal atresia is diagnosed by seeing a double bubble in the fetal stomach. Exomphalos is a defect in the anterior abdominal wall with the bowel and/or liver visible in a sac outside the body of the fetus. Renal agenesis is usually associated with anhydramnios which raises the suspicion of the ultrasonographer so that she/he carefully looks for the presence of the kidneys and bladder. Tracheoesophageal fistulae are only occasionally detected on ultrasound. Major cardiac abnormalities should be detected but the final diagnosis of the abnormality is usually made at 24 weeks from a detailed fetal cardiac ultrasound in a specialist unit.

2.21 ABDE

There are multiple causes of abdominal pain in pregnancy which include all causes that can occur outside pregnancy.

2.22 ABDGI

Women with pre-eclampsia should be delivered vaginally if at all possible. They are more likely to end up with a Caesarean section but they do not have to be delivered by Caesarean section. Epigastric pain is a symptom of hepatic capsule oedema and impending liver abnormalities as part of HELLP syndrome. Pre-eclampsia is associated with an increased risk of deep vein thrombosis and disseminated intravascular coagulation as well as placental abruption. Pre-eclampsia most commonly arises after 36 weeks of pregnancy. Magnesium sulphate is used in fulminating pre-eclampsia when there is a risk that the woman may develop eclampsia. First line treatment for hypertension includes methyldopa, hydralazine and nifedipine. Oedema is often present in pre-eclampsia but is not diagnostic.

2.23 ABC
Most women have a physiological anaemia in pregnancy due to an increased circulating plasma volume. The normal range in pregnancy is 10.5–12.5 g/dl. Below this value iron supplements should be offered, a transfusion is not warranted at term unless the woman is symptomatic which is very rare at an Hb of less than 10 g/dl and greater than 8 g/dl. Systemic iron is more appropriate but some women have an anaphylactic reaction to intramuscular iron. B_{12} deficiency is very rare in pregnancy and is usually secondary to excess alcohol intake or a pathological cause. Sickle cell disease and beta thalassaemia are both associated with anaemia in pregnancy.

2.24 C
There is no evidence that bed rest reduces the risk of miscarriage. Smoking is associated with IUGR.

2.25 E
Routine anomaly scanning should detect 100% of fetuses with anencephaly and up to 92% of spina bifida cases. The prognosis in spina bifida depends on the level and length of the defect. Fetuses with a spina bifida at L4/5 have a very high chance of survival into adult life although they may be incontinent and have partial lower limb paralysis. Pre-conceptual folic acid has been shown to significantly reduce the risk of neural tube defects.

2.26 C
All women who are rhesus negative should be given 500 IU Anti D if they have an antepartum haemorrhage. They do not require a transfusion unless the blood loss is significant and they are very anaemic.

2.27 E
Placenta praevia usually presents with painless vaginal bleeding. Placenta accreta, increta and percreta are terms which define the depth of invasion of the placenta into the myometrium.

2.28   BE
This woman is probably having a placental abruption and may go into shock. She should have a full blood count and cross match of two units of blood. Peripheral venous access is essential and 500 ml of Gelofusine (not normal saline) should be infused to maintain her intravascular circulating volume until blood is available. A cardiotocograph is indicated immediately to determine whether or not the baby is alive or is showing signs of hypoxia. A CVP may be needed later but is not the first line of action.

2.29   C
The Bishop's score is used to assess the cervix prior to induction of labour. The score determines the method of induction of labour.

2.30   ABC
10% of pregnancies present by the breech at less than 32 weeks. By term this has reduced to 2–3% because of spontaneous cephalic version.

2.31   DE
Breast feeding has been shown to increase the risk of vertical transmission of HIV from mother to baby. Antiretroviral agents have not been shown to be teratogenic.

2.32   BC
There is no evidence that a RML episiotomy reduces the risk of 3rd degree tear. Midline 2nd degree tears have been shown to heal faster than episiotomies. Assisted vaginal deliveries with a ventouse can be performed without recourse to an episiotomy as the ventouse does not increase the diameter of the fetal head. An episiotomy does allow the baby to deliver faster in the presence of fetal distress. In a case of shoulder dystocia an episiotomy allows internal manipulation of the shoulders to expedite delivery although there is no evidence that it increases the chances of delivering the shoulders using MacRobert's manoevre or suprapubic pressure.

2.33   D
The most likely diagnosis and the one that must be excluded is obstetric cholestasis which is known to increase the risk of intrauterine death. The diagnosis is made on abnormal liver function tests and raised bile acid levels.

2.34   CDE
Colostrum in the first few days and breast milk contain active white cells, macrophages, IgA, IgG and lactoferrin which are all anti-infective agents which protect the baby during the early weeks and months of life from bacterial and viral infections. Breast feeding reduces the risk of breast cancer in later life while pregnancy reduces the risk of ovarian cancer.

2.35   ACDE
Smoking and anorexia are both associated with intra-uterine growth restriction leading to premature delivery for fetal reasons. Smoking is associated with an increased risk of spontaneous pre-term labour. Essential hypertension increases the risk of early onset pre-eclampsia leading to delivery for maternal reasons and is also associated with intrauterine growth restriction. Obesity is associated with an increased risk of developing gestational diabetes but not pre-term delivery.

2.36   C
Candidiasis can affect the pharynx and mouth but rarely causes oral or genital ulcers, a pyrexia or lymphadenopathy. Gonorrhoea can present with pyrexia but does not cause ulcers. Syphilis causes oral and genital ulcers with lymphadenopathy but does not cause a high fever. Trichomonas presents with vaginal discharge and no other symptoms

2.37   B
GSUI is caused by descent of the bladder neck below the levator ani sling when intra-abdominal pressure is increased (laughing, coughing, sneezing). DI presents with frequency and urgency, neurogenic bladders commonly present with retention/overflow incontinence, pyelonephritis presents with a pyrexia, frequency, loin pain, renal colic. Urinary tract infections present with frequency and dysuria.

2.38 AC
Benign teratomas are more common in women under the age of 25 than in older women. They have an increased risk of torsion but rarely rupture because they have a thickened capsule. They can be diagnosed on plain abdominal X-ray because they commonly contain teeth which are radio-opaque. They do not interfere with ovulation and so do not present with amenorrhoea.

2.39 D
Ovarian cysts in early pregnancy are usually physiological (corpus luteum) and are necessary for the continuance of the pregnancy. They usually resolve spontaneously in the second trimester.

2.40 ACD
Menorrhagia is defined as a blood loss of > 80 ml per menstrual cycle. Sterilisation does not cause heavy periods. Bleeding is comparable to the women whose spouses have vasectomy which suggests that the problem is perception of loss rather than true heavy menstruation.

2.41 C
Polycystic ovary syndrome accounts for 70% of anovulatory subfertility.

2.42 BC
Endometriosis classically causes cyclical abdominal pain and often dyspareunia. It rarely affects tubal function or ovulation although it is associated with subfertility.

2.43 1:B 2:D 3:J 4:A 5:G
Symptoms of endometriosis most commonly arise in the late luteal phase. In an ectopic pregnancy it is quite common for women to have some vaginal bleeding at around the expected time of menses even though they are pregnant. A positive pregnancy test with unilateral pelvic pain and cervical excitation is strongly suggestive of an ectopic pregnancy. Torsion of an ovarian cyst is commonly associated with nausea and vomiting as is appendicitis. The lack of cervical excitation and a pyrexia suggests appendicitis. Bilateral tenderness with a high temperature suggests pelvic inflammatory disease.

2.44 B
Platinum based drugs remain the first line treatment for ovarian cancer. Carboplatin is less nephrotoxic and neurotoxic than cisplatin and is now the platinum based drug of choice. In 2002 the National Institute of Clinical Excellence (NICE) recommended the addition of Taxol as a first line drug following large multi-centre randomized trials.

2.45 AD
Human papilloma virus RNA has been found in 80% of cases of cervical squamocarcinoma. Stage I and II disease is usually treated with surgery. Stage III disease is usually treated with radiotherapy since cervical squamocarcinoma is not very chemosensitive. Chemotherapy is sometimes used to debulk the tumour prior to surgery.

2.46 B
Progestogens are the most effective because endometrial carcinoma is oestrogen dependent. It also has minimal side effects compared to the other chemotherapeutic agents.

2.47 BD
Echogenic foci in a cyst are always considered pathological and removal is recommended. In a woman of 53 there is an increased risk of ovarian cancer while a woman of 23 is more likely to have a dermoid cyst.

2.48 DE
Urinary retention can occur in the first few days following a vaginal hysterectomy but is not a recognized long-term complication.

2.49 AD
C and E would be considered reasons for a social termination or termination on demand, neither of which is legal in the UK. Over 24 weeks the fetus can be terminated if there is certain evidence that its condition would lead to a significant disability or death. If the baby needs to be delivered in order to save the mother's life as in fulminating pre-eclampsia or significant haemorrhage then induction of labour is appropriate but does not come under the terms of the Abortion Act 1967.

2.50   D

This is the treatment of choice for endometrial carcinoma stage I and II. Wertheim's hysterectomy is a radical hysterectomy which includes lymphadenectomy and is the treatment of choice in cervical cancer stage Ib.

PRACTICE PAPER 3

50 questions: Time allowed 2 hours.
Mark your answer with a tick (True) or a cross (False).
Do not look at the answers until you have completed the whole paper.
Answers and teaching notes are on page 83.

PRACTICE PAPER 3

3.1   Concerning the pelvis

☐ A   the transverse diameter of the pelvis averages 13 cm
☐ B   the longest axis of the pelvis rotates through 120°
        from top to bottom
☐ C   it is made up of three bones – two iliac bones and the
        sacrum
☐ D   the levator ani and the coccygeus muscle form the
        pelvic diaphragm
☐ E   the outlet of the pelvis has equal antero-posterior and
        transverse diameters

3.2   Choose from the following five statements best matched about gonadotrophin releasing hormone (GnRH):

☐ A   GnRH is produced by the thalamus
☐ B   GnRH is a small polypeptide
☐ C   GnRH inhibits the secretion of FSH
☐ D   GnRH is released continuously
☐ E   GnRH secretion is inhibited in women who are
        significantly obese
☐ F   GnRH secretion is inhibited by feedback of oestrogen
        and progesterone from the ovary
☐ G   GnRH is released into the pituitary portal system
☐ H   GnRH agonists are used to treat benign gynaecological
        disease
☐ I   GnRH agonists are used to treat malignant
        gynaecological disease
☐ J   GnRH secretion is inhibited in women who are
        significantly underweight

3.3   Which of the following statements are true?

☐ A   Oestrogens increase the vaginal pH by the action of
        Doderlein's bacillus on glycogen
☐ B   Progesterone increases the growth of the myometrium
        in pregnancy
☐ C   Progesterone increases the motility of the fallopian tubes
☐ D   Oestrogens increase the contractility of the myometrium
☐ E   Oestrogen reduces the viscosity of cervical mucus

3.4   Concerning the lymphatic drainage of the pelvis

❑ A   the vulva drains predominantly to the inguinal nodes
❑ B   the cervix drains predominantly to the internal iliac nodes
❑ C   the uterus drains predominantly to the external iliac nodes
❑ D   the cervix drains predominantly to the inguinal nodes
❑ E   the uterus drains predominantly to the para-aortic nodes

3.5   The transformation zone of the cervix

❑ A   is covered by columnar epithelium
❑ B   normally extends into the vaginal fornices
❑ C   forms in the second month of fetal development
❑ D   is histologically described as adenosis
❑ E   develops through the process of squamous metaplasia

3.6   Concerning fertilisation and implantation

❑ A   a single spermatozoon penetrates the polar body
❑ B   fertilisation occurs in the isthmus of the fallopian tube
❑ C   after fertilisation the endometrium swells and becomes the decidua of pregnancy
❑ D   implantation occurs about 12–14 days after fertilisation
❑ E   progesterone secretion from the endometrium is essential for successful implantation

3.7   Which of the following statements are true?

❑ A   The umbilical cord contains two veins and one artery
❑ B   The fetal surface of the placenta is covered by the chorion
❑ C   Amniotic fluid arises from the amniotic membrane and fetal urine
❑ D   Maternal blood flow to the uterus is 100–150 ml/kg/min in late pregnancy
❑ E   Oxygenated blood is carried directly into the left side of the fetal heart via the ductus arteriosus

3.8   Excessive vaginal discharge

❑ A   can be normal during the premenstrual phase
❑ B   is usually thick and white around the time of ovulation
❑ C   is always associated with vaginal infection
❑ D   can be confused with spontaneous rupture of
         membranes during pregnancy
❑ E   is commonly present in genital malignancy

3.9   Oestradiol

❑ A   is the principal hormone secreted by the developing
         follicle
❑ B   is secreted by the pituitary gland
❑ C   controls the proliferation of the endometrium
❑ D   controls the growth of the corpus luteum
❑ E   concentrations are highest at the onset of
         menstruation

3.10   Match five of the following infectious agents to the five statements below

A   Bacterial vaginosis
B   β-haemolytic streptococcus
C   Candida
D   Chlamydia
E   Gonorrhoea
F   Human immunodeficiency virus
G   *Staphylococcus aureus*
H   Syphilis
I   Trichomonas
J   Tuberculosis

❑ 1   is an organism which produces mycellae and spores
❑ 2   can be detected with dark field microscopy
❑ 3   is an organism which is flagellate
❑ 4   is found as a normal commensal in 10% of women
❑ 5   is detected on a smear by the presence of vaginal
         epithelial cells with a stippled cytoplasm

3.11 **Which one of the following tumour markers is most commonly used in the detection of epithelial ovarian cancer?**

- ❏ A LDH
- ❏ B hCG
- ❏ C AFP
- ❏ D CA125
- ❏ E CEA

3.12 **Which of the following statements are true of maternal changes in pregnancy?**

- ❏ A The red cell mass is increased
- ❏ B The red cell mass is decreased
- ❏ C The renal threshold for glucose is decreased
- ❏ D The renal reabsorption is increased by 50–60%
- ❏ E The renal threshold for glucose increases

3.13 **Concerning the menopause**

- ❏ A women who have not had a period for nine months are said to be postmenopausal
- ❏ B women who are postmenopausal may complain of urinary frequency and dysuria with a negative mid-stream urine culture
- ❏ C women who are postmenopausal may complain of dyspareunia because of vaginal constriction
- ❏ D women may experience periodic heavy vaginal bleeding round the time of the menopause
- ❏ E luteinising hormone levels rise before FSH levels as a woman becomes menopausal

3.14 For autosomal trisomy births

☐ A the risk of an autosomal trisomy increases with the gestational age of the fetus

☐ B the risk of Down's syndrome is lower than that for all trisomies regardless of maternal age

☐ C the risk of autosomal trisomy increases with the age of the father of the baby

☐ D the risk of autosomal trisomy increases with the age of the mother of the baby

☐ E the risk of an autosomal trisomy decreases with the gestational age of the fetus

3.15 Match A–E to five of the statements below

A A raised maternal α-fetoprotein concentration
B For positive hepatitis B serology
C Rubella infection in the 2nd trimester
D Rhesus negative women
E Toxoplasmosis serology testing

☐ 1 BCG immunization should be given to the neonate
☐ 2 is associated with deafness, blindness and mental retardation
☐ 3 is associated with macrosomia
☐ 4 identifies a group at high risk of fetal neural tube defect
☐ 5 Hep B immunization should be given to the neonate
☐ 6 is associated with an increased risk of cardiac abnormalities
☐ 7 is associated with an increased risk of Down's syndrome
☐ 8 should be offered to women who keep cats as pets
☐ 9 should be offered anti-D if they present with antepartum haemorrhage
☐ 10 should be offered to women who keep dogs as pets

3.16 Amniocentesis should be offered to all women

- ❏ A over the age of 32
- ❏ B with a positive Down's syndrome screening test
- ❏ C having their fourth child
- ❏ D with a family history of haemophilia
- ❏ E suspected of having a baby with a neural tube defect (NTD)

3.17 Fetal hypoxia in the antenatal period can be assessed by

- ❏ A fetal (Cardiff) kick chart
- ❏ B amniocentesis
- ❏ C liquor volume/amniotic fluid index
- ❏ D umbilical artery Doppler waveforms
- ❏ E abdominal palpation

3.18 Ultrasound measurement of the fetal abdominal circumference

- ❏ A gives an accurate estimated fetal weight at < 36 weeks gestation
- ❏ B accurately predicts shoulder dystocia
- ❏ C may be increased in women with gestational diabetes
- ❏ D is a good predictor of premature labour
- ❏ E may be increased in women with pre-eclampsia

3.19 Which of the following identify a woman at increased risk of developing maternal complications of pregnancy?

- ❏ A Age < 19
- ❏ B Past surgical history of appendicectomy
- ❏ C Multiple pregnancy
- ❏ D First degree relative with type 2 diabetes mellitus
- ❏ E First degree relative with type 1 diabetes
- ❏ F Age 20–34
- ❏ G Essential hypertension at booking
- ❏ H Sickle cell trait in the father of the baby
- ❏ I Low body mass index
- ❏ J Family history of Huntington's chorea

3.20 Which of the following statements are true?

❏ A Cardiac anomaly is the commonest fetal congenital abnormality
❏ B Cardiac anomalies affect 0.4–1.1% of live births
❏ C Fetal echocardiography is needed to make an accurate diagnosis
❏ D Cardiac anomaly is associated with a low nuchal translucency measurement
❏ E Routine anomaly ultrasound scans detect 90% of serious cardiac anomalies

3.21 Bilateral renal agenesis

❏ A occurs in 1:100,000 births
❏ B causes death within a few hours of birth
❏ C is associated with polyhydramnios
❏ D is an autosomal recessive disorder
❏ E is a common feature of babies with trisomy 21

3.22 A 26-year-old primigravid woman at ten weeks gestation visits her midwife for a routine booking appointment. She has sickle cell anaemia. Her partner's sickle cell status is HbAS. Her haemoglobin is 9.2 g/dl. What is the most appropriate management of this patient?

❏ A Genetic counselling
❏ B Penicillin
❏ C Hydroxyurea
❏ D IV hydration
❏ E Blood transfusion

3.23 Causes of spontaneous vaginal bleeding in pregnancy include

❏ A β haemolytic streptococci detected on a high vaginal swab
❏ B cervical polyp
❏ C preterm premature rupture of the membranes
❏ D cervical intraepithelial neoplasia grade 1
❏ E bacterial vaginosis

3.24 **A 34-year-old woman in her first pregnancy is admitted at term and three days in spontaneous labour. She is 4 cm dilated at 20.00 and is re-examined at 02.00 and found to be 4 cm dilated. The fetal heart rate is normal and the membranes are intact. Which of the following is the most appropriate action to take?**

❏ A Fetal blood sampling
❏ B Start a Syntocinon infusion
❏ C Perform a membrane sweep
❏ D Give Prostin 1 mg
❏ E Perform an artificial rupture of membranes

3.25 **Which of the following statements are true of induction of labour at term with intact membranes in a woman who has had an uncomplicated pregnancy?**

❏ A Prostin 1 mg can be used to induce labour
❏ B Misoprostol can be used to induce labour
❏ C Syntocinon can be used to induce labour
❏ D Artificial rupture of membranes can be used to induce labour
❏ E Mifepristone and misoprostol are used to induce labour

3.26 **Vaginal breech delivery can be considered in**

❏ A a primigravid woman at 42 weeks with a Bishop's score of 2
❏ B extended breech in spontaneous labour at term in an uncomplicated pregnancy
❏ C flexed breech in spontaneous labour at less than 36 weeks
❏ D footling breech in spontaneous labour at term in an uncomplicated pregnancy
❏ E footling breech in spontaneous labour at less than 36 weeks

3.27 Symptoms of postnatal depression include

- ❏ A insomnia
- ❏ B nausea
- ❏ C hyperactivity
- ❏ D anxiety
- ❏ E confusion

3.28 Antenatal steroid administration

- ❏ A is contraindicated in women with preterm premature rupture of the membranes
- ❏ B is recommended for all women in labour at less than 37 completed weeks of gestation
- ❏ C reduces the risk of neonatal intraventricular haemorrhage
- ❏ D is recommended for all women in labour at less than 34 completed weeks of gestation
- ❏ E should be given to all women with preterm premature rupture of the membranes

3.29 A woman presents at 34 weeks gestation complaining of itching. Her pregnancy is otherwise uncomplicated. The most likely diagnosis is

- ❏ A obstetric cholelithiasis
- ❏ B obstetric jaundice
- ❏ C obstetric cholestasis
- ❏ D obstetric eczema
- ❏ E obstetric psoriasis

3.30 A healthy term baby is born and at one minute shows no signs of breathing. The baby's heart rate is over 100 but the skin colour is blue and the baby is not moving. The most appropriate action to take is

- ❏ A suction to airways
- ❏ B cardiac massage
- ❏ C wrap the baby in a towel
- ❏ D give five breaths of oxygen via a face mask
- ❏ E intubate the baby

3.31 **Which of the following changes to obstetric practice have occurred following the reports of the Confidential Enquiries into maternal deaths over the last six years?**

- ❑ A Introduction of universal antenatal HIV screening
- ❑ B Consultant sessions on the labour ward
- ❑ C Routine thromboprophylaxis post Caesarean section
- ❑ D Routine antibiotic administration at the time of Caesarean section
- ❑ E Increased antenatal care in the community

3.32 **A 22-year-old woman visits her GP seeking advice for emergency contraception following intercourse 24 hours ago. She is very concerned that she may become pregnant. A urine pregnancy test is negative. Which of the following can be offered?**

- ❑ A Clomiphene
- ❑ B Combined pill
- ❑ C IUCD
- ❑ D Levonorgestrel
- ❑ E Danazol

3.33 **Concerning the vulva**

- ❑ A the clitoris is anterior to the urethra
- ❑ B the labia minora arise from the hood of the clitoris
- ❑ C the vestibule is the area between the anus and the vaginal introitus
- ❑ D the vestibule is the area from the perineal skin to the vaginal epithelium
- ❑ E the labia majora are equivalent to the penis in the male

3.34 **A 62-year-old woman attends her GP's surgery with vaginal itching and discomfort. Pelvic examination reveals a dry atrophic vagina with a thick white curd-like discharge. The most appropriate first line of management is**

- ❏ A clotrimazole vaginal cream
- ❏ B oestrogen vaginal cream
- ❏ C metronidazole vaginal cream
- ❏ D oral fluconazole
- ❏ E oral metronidazole

3.35 **A 20-year-old has her menstrual period every 45–60 days and lasts for five days with heavy blood loss. She was put on depot medroxyprogesterone acetate (Depo-Provera) for two years from age 17 to 19. During the second year she had no menstrual periods. Her menarche was at age 12. She suffered from acne to the age of 17. Which of the following is the abnormal pattern?**

- ❏ A Her cycle lasts 45–60 days
- ❏ B Her menses lasts five days
- ❏ C She suffered from acne to the age of 17
- ❏ D Menarche was at age 12
- ❏ E She had no menses for one year on DMPA

3.36 **A 15-year-old girl complains of cyclical pelvic pain each month. She has never had a menstrual period. Pelvic examination demonstrates a vaginal bulge. Urine pregnancy test is negative. Which of the following is the most likely diagnosis?**

- ❏ A Haematocolpos
- ❏ B Bicornuate uterus
- ❏ C Endometriosis
- ❏ D Imperforate hymen
- ❏ E Dermoid cyst

3.37 Which of the following are recognized as effective first or second line treatment of dysfunctional uterine bleeding?

❑ A Non-steroidal anti-inflammatory drugs (NSAIDs)
❑ B Cyclical progestogens
❑ C Antifibrinolytics
❑ D Progestogen only pill
❑ E Combined oral contraceptive pill

3.38 Which of the following conditions are associated with a raised follicle stimulating hormone (FSH)?

❑ A Hypogonadotrophic hypogonadism
❑ B Turner's syndrome
❑ C Polycystic ovary syndrome
❑ D Androgen insensitivity syndrome
❑ E Asherman's syndrome

3.39 For each condition (A–E) mark the first line treatment that gives the best chance of pregnancy:

A Anovulatory polycystic ovary syndrome
B Bilateral hydrosalpinges
C Hypogonadotrophic hypogonadism
D Klinefelter's syndrome
E Sperm count of < 0.2 x 10^6/ml

❑ 1   Egg donation
❑ 2   Donor insemination
❑ 3   Bromocriptine
❑ 4   Tubal surgery
❑ 5   Clomifene
❑ 6   Metformin
❑ 7   In-vitro fertilisation
❑ 8   Intracytoplasmic sperm injection (ICSI)
❑ 9   Follicle stimulating hormone
❑ 10 Preimplantation genetic diagnosis

3.40 Concerning hysterectomy

❏ A   a small number of women experience psychosexual problems following hysterectomy
❏ B   it guarantees a cure for menorrhagia
❏ C   it guarantees a cure for endometriosis
❏ D   it should be routinely offered to women with dysfunctional uterine bleeding
❏ E   most women have reported a high level of satisfaction with this operation

3.41 A 58-year-old woman presents with a unilateral ovarian cyst accompanied by a large omental metastasis. Which one of the following is the surgical treatment of choice?

❏ A   Total abdominal hysterectomy and bilateral salpingo-oophorectomy
❏ B   Total abdominal hysterectomy and unilateral oophorectomy
❏ C   Excision of the omental metastasis and unilateral oophorectomy
❏ D   Omentectomy and bilateral salpingo-oophorectomy
❏ E   Omentectomy, total abdominal hysterectomy, and bilateral salpingo-oophorectomy

3.42 A 72-year-old woman presents with four episodes of post-menopausal bleeding over the last six months. She is otherwise fit and well although her BMI is 38 kg/m^2. What investigations should be performed to determine the diagnosis?

❏ A   Hysteroscopy alone
❏ B   Examination under anaesthesia, hysteroscopy and endometrial biopsy
❏ C   Transvaginal ultrasound scan and outpatient endometrial biopsy
❏ D   Vaginal examination and outpatient endometrial biopsy
❏ E   MRI scan and outpatient endometrial biopsy

3.43 Which of the following statements accurately describes a Wertheim's hysterectomy?

❏ A Hysterectomy and bilateral salpingo-oophorectomy
❏ B Hysterectomy and bilateral salpingo-oophorectomy and inguinal lymphadenectomy
❏ C Hysterectomy and bilateral salpingo-oophorectomy, internal, external iliac and obturator lymphadenectomy
❏ D Hysterectomy and bilateral salpingo-oophorectomy, internal, external iliac and inguinal lymphadenectomy
❏ E Hysterectomy and bilateral salpingo-oophorectomy, internal, external iliac and para-aortic lymphadenectomy

3.44 A 76-year-old woman presents with a 2 cm unilateral, invasive vulvar carcinoma with no evidence of lymph node involvement. The recommended management is

❏ A simple vulvectomy and bilateral inguinal lymphadenectomy
❏ B radiation therapy
❏ C simple vulvectomy
❏ D chemotherapy
❏ E wide local excision

3.45 Which of the following are ovarian germ cell tumours?

❏ A Dysgerminoma
❏ B Granulosa cell tumour
❏ C Dermoid cyst
❏ D Epithelial cell tumour
❏ E Mucinous cystadenocarcinoma

3.46 Risk factors for development of acute pelvic inflammatory disease include

❏ A aged 15 to 24 years
❏ B oral contraceptives
❏ C presence of an intrauterine device
❏ D multiple sexual partners
❏ E barrier contraception

3.47 Risk of failure of the oral contraceptive pill can be significantly increased by

- ❏ A breakthrough bleeding on days 12–14 of calendar pack
- ❏ B missing three pills on days 12–14 of the calendar pack
- ❏ C missing three pills on days 19–21 of the calendar pack
- ❏ D missing three pills on days 4–6 of the calendar pack
- ❏ E concurrent taking of antibiotics

3.48 Absolute contraindications to the use of the combined oral contraceptive pill include

- ❏ A family history of breast cancer
- ❏ B essential hypertension
- ❏ C epilepsy
- ❏ D headaches
- ❏ E warfarin therapy

3.49 Regarding miscarriage

- ❏ A the commonest cause of sporadic miscarriage is a chromosomal abnormality
- ❏ B the outcome of pregnancy in women with antiphospholipid syndrome is significantly improved with aspirin and warfarin
- ❏ C the commonest cause of sporadic miscarriage is antiphospholipid syndrome
- ❏ D the risk of miscarriage increases with age
- ❏ E the outcome of pregnancy in women with antiphospholipid syndrome is significantly improved with aspirin and heparin

3.50 Concerning the fetal skull

- ❏ A it has two membranous areas which are diamond shaped
- ❏ B the suboccipitofrontal diameter is the largest presenting diameter
- ❏ C the vertex is presentation by the submentobregmatic diameter
- ❏ D the vertex is presentation by the mentovertical diameter
- ❏ E the vertex is presentation by the suboccipitobregmatic diameter

3.1	ACD		3.26	BC
3.2	BFGHJ		3.27	AD
3.3	BDE		3.28	BCE
3.4	AB		3.29	C
3.5	E		3.30	D
3.6	CE		3.31	BCD
3.7	CD		3.32	CD
3.8	AD		3.33	ABD
3.9	AC		3.34	A
3.10	1:C 2:H 3:I 4:B 5:A		3.35	A
3.11	D		3.36	D
3.12	AC		3.37	ACE
3.13	BD		3.38	BD
3.14	BDE		3.39	A:5 B:7 C:9 D:2 E:8
3.15	A:4 B:5 C:2 D:9 E:8		3.40	ABE
3.16	BE		3.41	E
3.17	ACD		3.42	B
3.18	AC		3.43	C
3.19	ACDGI		3.44	A
3.20	ABC		3.45	AC
3.21	B		3.46	CD
3.22	A		3.47	CDE
3.23	B		3.48	BE
3.24	E		3.49	ADE
3.25	ABD		3.50	E

PAPER 3 – ANSWERS AND TEACHING NOTES

3.1   ACD
The longest axis of the pelvis rotates through 90º not 120º. The outlet of the pelvis is diamond shaped with its longest axis running antero-posteriorly.

3.2   BFGHJ
GnRH is a small polypeptide produced by the hypothalamus. It flows through the pituitary portal system to stimulate the secretion of LH and FSH from the pituitary gland. GnRH is released in pulses every 90 minutes and this pulsatile secretion is vital for continued reproductive function. Continuous GnRH secretion leads to decreased stimulation of the pituitary. Because of this GnRH agonist is used in the treatment of benign gynaecological disease such as endometriosis. The secretion of GnRH is controlled by feedback of estrogen and progesterone from the ovary.

3.3   BDE
Doderlein's bacilli reduce the pH of the vaginal secretions. Oestrogen and progesterone both reduce the motility of the fallopian tube. Progesterone reduces the contractility of the myometrium whilst oestrogen increases it. Oestrogen reduces the viscosity of cervical and vaginal secretions in order to allow sperm to travel more easily into the uterus.

3.4   AB
The uterus drains predominantly to the internal iliac nodes.

3.5   E
The transformation zone is formed by squamous metaplasia of columnar cells that line the cervical canal. Usually the transformation zone lies just inside the cervical canal. Under the influence of oestrogens (in pregnancy or if the woman is on the combined oral contraceptive pill) the transformation zone extends onto the surface of the cervix (an ectropion) but never into the vaginal fornices.

Paper 3 – Answers and Teaching Notes

3.6　CE
Fertilisation usually takes place in the ampullary region of the fallopian tube. A single spermatozoon penetrates the zona pellucida of the oocyte not the polar body which regresses soon after fertilisation. The embryo implants between six and eight days after fertilisation. Progesterone is essential for the changes in the arterioles and glands of the uterus to produce spiraling and secretion of glycogen for the nutrition of the developing embryo in the tube and uterus. Decidualisation of the endometrium is also controlled by progesterone and mucopolysaccharides secreted on the surface of the embryo.

3.7　CD
The umbilical cord contains two arteries and one vein. The fetal surface of the placenta is covered by the amnion – the chorion is fused at the edges of the placental disc. Oxygenated blood is carried along the umbilical artery into the right side of the heart and on to the left side through the foramen ovale. In order to prevent pulmonary hypertension the ductus arteriosus runs between the pulmonary artery and the aorta so that only a small amount of oxygenated blood from the right side of the heart reaches the pulmonary circulation.

3.8　AD
Vaginal discharge changes throughout the menstrual cycle. In the early follicular and late luteal phase there is often very little discharge which, if present is usually thick and white. Mid-cycle the discharge becomes less viscid and acellular allowing the sperm to flow through more easily. In the luteal phase the discharge is usually thick and creamy white.

3.9　AC
Oestroadiol is the main steroid hormone secreted by the developing follicle. It controls the growth of the endometrium in the follicular phase of the cycle mainly by increasing the number of cells (proliferation). Secretion of estrogen is controlled by LH and FSH. Estrogen levels are at their lowest premenstrually and their highest at the time of ovulation.

84

3.10   1:C 2:H 3:I 4:B 5:A

Bacterial vaginosis/Gardnerella are commonly associated with clue cells (vaginal epithelial cells with a stippled cytoplasm). Tuberculosis is a mycobacterium and may rarely cause pelvic inflammatory disease. Chlamydia is detected using an enzyme linked immunoassay or fluorescent monoclonal antibodies on a smear. Gonorrhoea is a Gram positive coccus which grows in Stewarts medium. Spirochaetes can be detected by dark field microscopy in primary syphilis whilst serum tests are used to detect secondary syphilis. *Staph. aureus* is a common commensal on the skin which may cause toxic shock syndrome if the vagina becomes infected.

3.11   D

LDH, hCG, AFP are all associated with choriocarcinoma, teratomas and dysgerminomas. CEA is most commonly used in the detection of gastric and colonic tumours.

3.12   AC

The red cell mass is increased but there is a relative anaemia because of the increased plasma volume. The renal threshold for glucose is decreased so it is more common to find glucose in the urine of pregnant women even if they are not diabetic. The renal reabsorption is increased by 30–50%.

3.13   BD

A woman is defined as being postmenopausal if she has not had a period for 12 months. Withdrawal of oestrogen causes changes to the urethral and vaginal epithelium causing dryness, irritation and dyspareunia. Heavy irregular vaginal bleeding is quite common around the time of the menopause because the endometrium is exposed to oestrogens, even though the ovaries are no longer ovulating. FSH levels rise before LH levels.

3.14   BDE

Trisomy is a recognized cause of spontaneous miscarriage so with increasing gestation the risk of trisomy decreases with increasing gestational age of the fetus. Down's syndrome is only one of the trisomies so the risk for all trisomies is greater at all ages. The age of the father does not seem to increase the risk of trisomy.

3.15   A:4 B:5 C:2 D:9 E:8

Serum α-fetoprotein concentrations are raised in normal pregnancy but are often significantly raised in women who have a fetus with a neural tube defect and reduced in a Down's syndrome pregnancy. Hepatitis B is rarely transmitted to the fetus in-utero but may be in the immediate neonatal period so immunisation is recommended for neonates born to hepatitis B positive mothers. Toxoplasmosis can cause fetal mental retardation, IUGR and intrauterine death and is transmitted from the faeces of cats – so women are advised not to handle cat litter trays. Dog faeces can cause trachoma in young children. Rubella infection in the 2nd trimester is associated with deafness, blindness and mental retardation. Cardiac abnormalities are associated with the major trisomies and there is an increased risk in women with poorly controlled type 1 diabetes. Gestational diabetes is associated with macrosomia.

3.16   BE

The risk of Down's syndrome starts to rise from the age of 36 at conception, at 32 the risk from age alone is around 1:600. The risk of Down's syndrome does not increase with the number of pregnancies, although many women having their fourth child may be over the age of 36. Women with a family history of haemophilia are usually offered chorionic villous sampling because this can be performed earlier and it is easier to do PCR on a CVS sample than from the squames obtained at amniocentesis. An amniocentesis can be used if a NTD is suspected for the measurement of α-fetoprotein rather than chromosomes since NTDs are rarely associated with a chromosomal abnormality.

3.17 ACD
Fetal movements are a good indicator of fetal well-being. The Cardiff kick chart asks women to mark the time each day when they have felt the baby kick ten times. A reduction in liquor volume is an indication that the baby may be becoming hypoxic and is often associated with intrauterine growth restriction (IUGR). Umbilical artery waveforms are used to detect fetuses which are hypoxic. Absent end diastolic flow and reverse end diastolic flow are signs that the fetus is probably becoming hypoxic. Amniocentesis is used to detect chromosomal abnormalities, infection, jaundice secondary to haemolytic disease of the newborn and rarely these days to see if the lungs are mature using the lecithin:sphingomyelin ratio. It is not used to detect hypoxia. Abdominal palpation is relatively poor at detecting IUGR and, unless fetal movements are felt, is not a good measure of fetal well-being.

3.18 AC
Measurement of fetal abdominal circumference does not accurately predict shoulder dystocia although it can identify a group of babies that are at increased risk. The fetal AC is used to detect macrosomia in gestational diabetics and IUGR in women with pre-eclampsia where the AC may be reduced relative to the head circumference.

3.19 ACDGI
Teenage pregnancies have an increased prevalence of pre-eclampsia or pregnancy induced hypertension compared with women aged 20–34. A first degree relative with type 2 diabetes increases the risk of the mother developing gestational diabetes (GDM) because the family may have a genetic predisposition to insulin resistance. A first degree relative with type 1 diabetes does not increase the risk of developing complications in pregnancy. Essential hypertension at booking increases the risk of developing pre-eclampsia (PET). Multiple pregnancy increases the risk of complications in pregnancy, particularly GDM and PET. Women with a low BMI are at increased risk of having a small for gestational age baby. Sickle cell trait in either parent or a family history of Huntington's chorea does not increase the risk of maternal complications although genetic counselling with regard to the risk of the fetus inheriting sickle cell anaemia or Huntington's chorea should be offered.

3.20   ABC
Cardiac anomalies are associated with an increased nuchal translucency measurement because of early onset fetal hydrops. Routine anomaly ultrasound scans detect 40–61% of serious cardiac anomalies. Fetal cardiac echocardiography is required for an accurate diagnosis.

3.21   B
Renal agenesis occurs in 1:3000–10,000 births. Recurrence rate is 2–5%. Unilateral agenesis is more common than bilateral agenesis. Renal agenesis is associated with early onset oligohydramnios and pulmonary hypoplasia. It is not an inherited disorder. It is a common feature of trisomy 16 and 13 but is virtually never seen in babies with Down's syndrome. Bilateral renal agenesis is universally fatal shortly after birth.

3.22   A
This woman does not have sickle cell disease so she does not require any medical intervention. Genetic counselling will inform her of the risk for her child having sickle cell anaemia so she can decide whether or not to have a chorionic villous sample test to establish whether the child has sickle cell anaemia or not.

3.23   B
β haemolytic streptococci are found as a normal commensal in 10% of women. CIN 1 does not cause spontaneous vaginal bleeding whilst a polyp may. Preterm premature rupture of the membranes is not a cause of vaginal bleeding unless there is placental abruption or placenta praevia associated with it.

3.24   E
After four hours one would expect the cervical dilatation to be 8 cm (1 cm/hour). Plotting the partogram would show that this woman had reached the action line. Since the membranes are intact the next action should be to rupture the membranes. A membrane sweep is performed if a woman has not gone into spontaneous labour at term plus 5–9 days to try and encourage onset (70% of women will go into spontaneous labour within 48 hours). Prostin is used to induce labour and is never used in active labour. Syntocinon should not be started with the membranes intact.

3.25 ABD
Mifepristone and misoprostol are used for medical terminations of pregnancy and for induction of labour in cases of intrauterine death (not normal) at any gestation. Misoprostol alone is being increasingly used for induction of labour because it is much cheaper than Prostin and as effective. Syntocinon alone should not be used if the membranes are intact. Artificial rupture of membranes is used if the cervix is already dilated (Bishop's score > 6) – most commonly in multigravid women.

3.26 BC
Vaginal breech delivery can be considered at term in a normally grown fetus presenting as an extended breech provided the onset of labour is spontaneous and progress in labour is normal. Induction of labour is contraindicated in breech presentations particularly when the cervix is found to be unfavourable for induction (Bishop's score < 4). The risks of fetal hypoxia and neonatal death are increased and the woman needs careful counselling. Footling breeches should be delivered by Caesarean section at all gestations because of the increased risk of cord prolapse and fetal head entrapment. Below 36 weeks there is no evidence that the outcome for the baby is worse in vaginal versus abdominal deliveries.

3.27 AD
Hyperactivity and confusion are symptoms of postnatal psychosis rather than depression. Nausea is not a symptom of postnatal depression and is rare in the postnatal period.

3.28 BCE
Although steroids increase the risk of infection the benefit of steroid administration for the fetus is much greater than the risk to the mother of sepsis and should therefore be given to all women in premature labour. The main benefits for the fetus are a reduction in the risk of developing severe respiratory distress syndrome and intraventricular haemorrhage. Recent guidelines from the Royal College of Obstetricians and Gynaecologists recommend that steroids should be given to all women in labour at less than 37 completed weeks of gestation.

3.29   C
The most likely diagnosis and the one that must be excluded is obstetric cholestasis which is known to increase the risk of intrauterine death. Eczema and psoriasis do cause itching but are usually present prior to pregnancy and are associated with well recognized rashes. Cholelithiasis and jaundice are rarely precipitated by pregnancy.

3.30   D
Suction to the airways causes bradycardia and unless there is thick meconium the priority is to give the baby oxygen via a mask. Five breaths from a 250 ml bag via a face mask is the recommended first step to clear fluid from the lungs. Cardiac massage is not indicated as the heart rate is greater than 100.

3.31   BCD
HIV testing is not universal yet in England and Wales but is highly recommended in areas with a high prevalence (inner cities). Early consultant involvement in high risk cases has been a recommendation in every Confidential Enquiry and has finally resulted in consultants being present during the day on the majority of labour wards. Thromboprophylaxis has been shown to reduce the incidence of post-partum thrombosis and antibiotics reduce the incidence of post-partum sepsis. Increased antenatal care in the community was recommended by Baroness Cumberledge but has yet to prove that it reduces maternal mortality.

3.32   CD
The aim of emergency contraception is to prevent implantation of a fertilized ovum. Clomiphene is used to induce ovulation. The combined pill when taken correctly prevents ovulation but does not prevent implantation of a fertilized ovum. Danazol is a progestogen and does not prevent implantation.

3.33   ABD
The labia majora are equivalent to the scrotal skin in the male. The clitoris is the penile equivalent in a female.

3.34 A

This woman has candidiasis as her primary diagnosis. A topical antifungal treatment is the treatment of choice. Oral antifungals are used as second or third line therapy.

3.35 A

The normal range for the duration of the menstrual cycle is 26–32 days. Acne is very common in teenagers. Following prolonged use of Depo-Provera amenorrhoea is common and it can take up to 18 months for ovulation to resume on a regular basis.

3.36 D

The history is suggestive of obstructed outflow of menstrual blood. Haematocolpos (secondary to cervical stenosis) is a very rare congenital abnormality whilst imperforate hymen is more common. Endometriosis, bicornuate uterus and dermoid cysts are not a cause of primary amenorrhoea.

3.37 ACE

Evidence shows that NSAIDs decrease the menstrual loss by 30% in women proven to have heavy periods. In contrast cyclical progestogens and the progestogen only pill have been shown to be ineffective. Antifibrinolytics (tranexamic acid) reduce blood loss by up to 40%. The combined oral contraceptive pill is highly effective in women with no contraindications.

3.38 BD

Turner's syndrome girls have streak gonads that do not produce estrogen or oocytes so there is no negative feedback on the pituitary. Women with PCOS may have a raised luteinising hormone but have normal FSH levels. Women with androgen insensitivity syndrome have normal male testosterone levels (unless they have had a gonadectomy) but have no ability to respond to testosterone so there is no negative feedback on the pituitary. If they have had a gonadectomy then the levels are raised as per Turner's syndrome.

3.39   A:5 B:7 C:9 D:2 E:8
Men with Klinefelter's cannot use their own sperm (if they have any) as there is a high risk of trisomy. Clomiphene achieves ovulation in 70% of women with PCOS. Women with hypogonadotrophic hypogonadism have a 90% chance of becoming pregnant with FSH injections. In vitro fertilisation has a higher success rate and lower ectopic pregnancy rate than tubal surgery for bilateral tubal damage. Intracytoplasmic sperm injection (ICSI) is successful as a treatment for oligospermia.

3.40   ABE
Endometriosis will not be cured by hysterectomy alone, removal of the ovaries is required as well. Since dysfunctional uterine bleeding is not associated with any pathology more conservative methods of treatment should be routinely offered before hysterectomy is performed.

3.41   E
Ovarian cysts should always be assumed to be malignant in post-menopausal women. An omental metastasis confirms the diagnosis of ovarian cancer. Surgery therefore includes removal of ovaries, tube, uterus and omentum.

3.42   B
This remains the staging procedure of choice because the examination will reveal any parametrial involvement which alters the stage of disease and subsequent therapy. More recently this procedure is being performed in outpatients under local anaesthetic. A formal endometrial biopsy is essential rather than an endometrial sample obtained using a pipelle or Vabra cannula.

3.43   C
Inguinal lymph nodes are removed in cases of vulval carcinoma and para-aortic nodes are biopsied in cases of ovarian carcinoma. In cervical carcinoma all pelvic lymph nodes are removed.

3.44 A
The lymphatic drainage of the vulva is to the inguinal nodes. Even if there is no clinical evidence of lymphatic involvement the inguinal nodes should be removed.

3.45 AC
Granulosa cell tumours secrete oestrogen. Mucinous cystadenoma is a benign epithelial cell ovarian cyst. Dermoid cysts contain well-differentiated embryonic tissues including teeth, bone, neural tissue, renal tissue etc.

3.46 CD
Although some young women tend to have more sexual partners age alone does not increase the risk per se. Oral contraceptives protect against pelvic inflammatory disease (PID) by thickening the vaginal secretions. Barrier contraception is the most effective preventive measure against PID.

3.47 CDE
Missing pills at the end of a packet or failing to start a new packet on time increases the pill free interval and allows the ovary to ovulate. Antibiotics can increase the gastrointestinal transit time and reduce absorption of the pill making it less effective.

3.48 BE
The combined oral contraceptive pill is associated with an increased risk of developing hypertension and thrombosis thus making these two pre-existing conditions absolute contra-indications for taking the combined oral contraceptive pill.

3.49 ADE
Warfarin is used to treat proven thromboembolic disease. The majority of women with recurrent miscarriage associated with antiphospholipid syndrome have not had a proven deep vein thrombosis or a pulmonary embolus. Warfarin is contra-indicated in the early stages of pregnancy so heparin is used in prophylactic doses. This has been shown to improve the take home baby rate from 10% to 40% in such women. Miscarriage is significantly more common in women aged over 38.

3.50   E
The two membranous areas are called fontanelles. The anterior one is diamond shaped whilst the posterior one is triangular. The largest diameter is the mentovertical diameter (brow presentation). The submentobregmatic diameter is a face presentation but has the same diameter as the suboccipito-bregmatic diameter (vertex presentation). The suboccipito-frontal diameter is only slightly larger than a vertex presentation and does not normally cause a problem.

INDEX

Index

Index

Index

BOOKS FOR MEDICAL STUDENTS FROM PASTEST

Essential MCQs for Medical Finals, Second edition
Rema Wasan, Delilah Hassanally,
Balvinder Wasan   ISBN 1 901198 20 0

Essential MCQs for Surgical Finals, Second edition
Delilah Hassanally, Rema Singh   ISBN 1 901198 15 4

Essential MCQs in Clinical Pharmacology
Delilah Hassanally, Rema Singh   ISBN 1 901198 32 4

EMQs for Medical Students Volume One
Adam Feather et al   ISBN 1 901198 65 0

EMQs for Medical Students Volume Two
Adam Feather et al   ISBN 1 901198 69 3

OSCEs for Medical Undergraduates Volume One
Adam Feather, Ramanathan Visvanathan,
John SP Lumley   ISBN 1 901198 04 9

OSCEs for Medical Undergraduates Volume Two
Ramanathan Visvanathan, Adam Feather,
John SP Lumley   ISBN 1 901198 05 7

Medical Finals: Passing the Clinical
Christopher Moore, Anne Richardson ISBN 1 901198 43 6

Surgical Finals: passing the Clinical, Second edition
John SP Lumley, Gina Kuperberg   ISBN 1 901198 77 4

Medical Finals: Structured Answers and Essay Questions
Adam Feather, Ramanathan Visvanathan,
John SP Lumley   ISBN 1 901198 79 7

Surgical Finals: Structured Answers and Essay Questions
Ramanathan Visvanathan,
John SP Lumley   ISBN 1 901198 43 X

Learning by Lists for Medical Students
Stuart McPherson   ISBN 1 901198 30 8

**The Practical Guide to Medical Ethics and Law for Junior
Doctors and Medical Students**
Chloe-Maryse Baxter, Mark Brennan,
Yvette Coldicott   ISBN 1 901198 76 6

Radiology Casebook for Medical Students
Rema Wasan, Alan Grundy, Richard Beese   ISBN 1 901198 40 5

Clinical Skills for Medical Students: A Hands-on Guide
Ian Bickle, David McCluskey, Barry Kelly   ISBN 1 901198 86 3